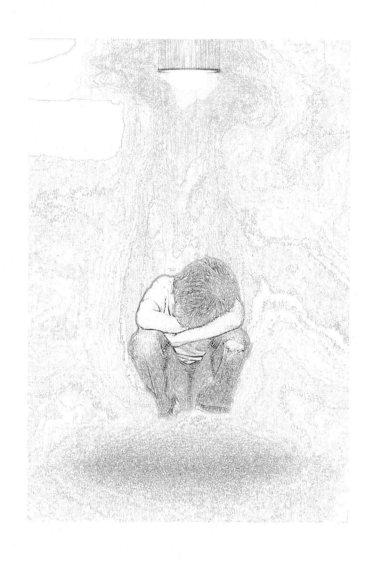

SHADOW SYNDROMES

Shining a Light on PANS and Other Inflammation-Based Illnesses Plaguing Today's Youth

Anymom

DISCLAIMER

No portion of this book is intended to offer medical or treatment advice, nor does this story reflect the medical or treatment advice of any medical providers. If you are facing a *Pediatric Autoimmune Neuropsychiatric Syndrome* (PANS) diagnosis, inform yourself in as many ways as possible. There are a multitude of books, websites, and social media sites that provide detailed and explicit information on the topic of PANS. May this book be one of many stepping-stones that you use on your journey back to peace and wellness for your child.

This is our story, one unique account of a devastating, poorly understood illness that has brought suffering to countless children and families the world over. Because PANS is an emerging illness and more research needs to be done, no portion of our story should be generalized or interpreted as representative of any child other than our own. In the telling of our story, we have touched on topics that physicians, researchers, and other Anyparents may find controversial: things like gluten intolerance, vaccination reactions, and methylation issues, to name a few. We have shared these things not because we are promoting a theory, implying causation, or seeking approval or conflict. We are simply sharing our story.

ACKNOWLEDGMENTS

Thank you to the doctors, nurses, and hospitals who, one-by-one, appeared on our horizon to begin leading us out of the dark fog that is PANS.

Jennifer Frankovich, MD, MS
Theresa A. Willett, MD, Ph.D
Margo Thienemann, MD
Jeanne Kane, MA
Kiki Chang, MD
Rosario Trifiletti, MD, Ph.D
Amy Fishman Smith, NP

Lucile Packard Children's Hospital Stanford
University of California Davis Children's Hospital
Stanford University

To the Stanford PANS Clinic: For the exemplary medical care you have given to Anychild and for renewing our faith in the compassion of medicine.

To my Anyparents and Extended Family and to our Anyfriends: You each took the time to learn about PANS, to try to comprehend it, so that you could better understand and love Anychild and our family while we took this horrid journey. On many days your love and support made all the difference.

To Anydad: Your integrity as a husband and a father is flawless. Thank you for your support, your trust, and your love.

To our three Anychildren: This book may be about one of you, but it is just a book. In life, in our family, and in my heart, there is no hierarchy. May you each know that you are infinitely loved, heard, and respected; and that the three of you walk on equal ground in our family. If there is one familial lesson that this journey through PANS has left me in possession of, it is the awareness of the destructive power invoked by giving one child in a family precedence above all others. As clear as my maternal intentions are, parenting is an imperfect art and if there is ever a time when I fail at this task of always offering *each one of you equal footing in our family*, please just say so—and I will do whatever I need to in order to fix it.

CREDITS DUE

There is a considerable amount of negative tension that occurs when on a journey with PANS. This negative tension, as uncomfortable as it is, can be a primary part of the growth process. Alchemy never occurs without heat and pressure, so the following credits are offered to those who provided both:

> To the Anydocs who looked at us with cool indifference while we searched desperately for ways to heal our son: You have taught us fortitude. We hope that someday the stories of Anyfamilies like us will teach you humility.

> And to the Anylookers who have judged and accused us: Your audacity paired with your ignorance made going forward with this book a necessity.

There are two ways of spreading light:
to be the candle or the
mirror that reflects it.
~Edith Wharton

This book is dedicated to the thousands of
Anyfamilies who are on their own in the
wilderness of PANDAS/PANS.

If you are new to this journey, may our story be
a candle . . . and one small part of what helps you
to build a bridge to high quality, informed medical
care for your Anychild.

If you are a seasoned Anyparent who has been on
the frontlines fighting for your Anychild, may our
story be a mirror that reflects your story and helps
raise awareness for all of us.

Together may we find a way to bring these shadow
syndromes that plague our children into the light
of day.

For every print copy of this book purchased 20% of the net proceeds will be donated to the Stanford PANS Clinic and Research Fund.

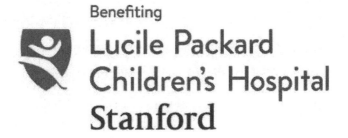

Benefiting

Lucile Packard
Children's Hospital
Stanford

PART ONE

We are Anyfamily. We live in Anytown, USA, where we are raising our little boy, who you will know as Anychild. This is a true story and we are a real family with real hopes and dreams. Our Anychild is a beautiful, blonde-haired, blue-eyed boy who has little dimples above his eyebrows and who never stops moving or asking why. Neither do we.

ANYCHILD

We have always called him "the caboose." As our third and final genetic contribution to the human race, Anychild was the late-in-life baby I had always hoped for. I still vividly remember the Labor and Delivery nurse's wry commentary on the day Anychild was born. As she expertly wrapped him in that burrito hold that all neonatal nurses are skilled at, she laughed and asked if I had a onesie for him that said, "Popsicles for Breakfast?"

When I raised an eyebrow at her query, she noted that with third children, all the hard and fast rules parents manage to stick to with their first two kids fall away in favor of mere survival.

At the time, I felt I was far too adept as a parent to ever feel as if I could "just survive" with my child. Little did I know. Perhaps it was this bold display of parental arrogance that first made the Fates look our way . . .

Other than arriving into the world a full pound heavier than either of his siblings had been at birth, there was nothing that set Anychild too far apart from what we had known with our other children— until he got his first ear infection just before his second birthday.

He had awakened inconsolable that morning. Although it was clear that something was wrong, because he had no fever, no rash, no outward symptoms of anything at all, we weren't sure what it was. Even so, it was clear that he was out of his head with discomfort due to *something*. Just the act of getting his flailing body into the car seat so we could drive to the pediatrician's office was a feat of epic proportions.

I struggled into the waiting room with him and took a seat to await our turn. He laid down at my feet and had a full on meltdown, and the more I tried to scoop him off the germ-filled floor, the harder and more violently he kicked and heaved himself at me. I was not used to being the mother of 'that kid,' and it is fair to say that I was more than a little bit mortified at the scene that was unfolding.

In an attempt to justify the ruckus we had created in the waiting room, I gamely explained to our pediatrician that over the preceding twenty-four hours, Anychild had been acting like a caged animal.

He nodded his head to affirm he was listening as he began to do a physical exam on Anychild. My caged animal reference was soon fully appreciated when Anychild displayed an enormous resistance to being touched.

When all was said and done, it took three of us—the doctor, his medical assistant, and myself—to wrestle Anychild into submission so that his ears, nose, throat, and belly could be checked. The only thing that this exam revealed was a slightly bulging ear-drum. The doctor supposed that it was infected, but he was utterly perplexed at the level of discomfort Anychild was displaying in light of this rather miniscule finding. He wrote a prescription for an antibiotic and based on Anychild's level of distress, he referred us to an Ear/Nose and Throat doctor.

We wasted no time following up on the referral. One mild ear infection had created a family-wide disturbance. After Anychild began the antibiotics and the infection cleared, it took weeks to get him settled back into a normal routine. It was humbling that a slightly bulging eardrum had turned our world upside down.

Humbling or not, in defense of never wanting to experience this again, Anychild was shortly thereafter scheduled for a myringotomy. Yes, just one slight ear infection and Anychild became the proud owner of a set of ear tubes. When I look back on the fact that we agreed to have surgery performed on our child just to make sure that he never again faced even a slight buildup of pressure behind his eardrums, I know now that was a clue we did not see.

The tubes did their job and Anychild never experienced another ear infection. For the majority of the three years that followed, he was robustly healthy. Only one other time did he get 'sick' in the proper sense of the word, and it was when he came down with what our pediatrician eventually deemed a case of Coxsackie B, also known as 'Hand, Foot, and Mouth disease.' Anychild had few outward signs of illness and never developed a fever. His main symptom was that he was highly distraught and very difficult to manage behaviorally.

What I most vividly remember about this bout of illness was what happened to Anychild's legs. During the course of the week-long virus, Anychild stopped walking. For three days straight he simply refused to bear any weight on his legs at all. He cried out in pain any time he attempted to stand and collapsed to the floor in a heap. The pediatrician felt that this was more behavioral than physical, as he could find no reason for such leg pain. Despite my silent disagreement with the notion that this was a behavioral issue for Anychild, there was little that I could do but trust our doctor's judgment and soldier on. Sure enough, within days the virus passed and Anychild's inability to walk passed with it.

Other than these two mild childhood illnesses—
an ear infection and a bout of Coxsackie B—Anychild
marched through childhood with nary a symptom of
any other childhood illness. There was never a runny
nose, no bright pink cheeks, or any other typical
childhood illnesses. As far as we could tell, Anychild
seemed to be a radiantly healthy child.

In retrospect, when I look at the unusual way the
two routine illnesses he did contract played out in his
immune system, it seems the writing was on the wall
. . . but we never knew that wall existed until we hit
it head on in February of 2012.

GAME CHANGER

It was an early winter morning, and I had taken
Anychild to the pediatrician for his 5-year-old 'well
child' exam. We had practiced a delayed vaccination
schedule up to this point, and at this exam he was
due for several shots. Without these inoculations, he
could not start kindergarten the following September,
and at the age of five, I felt that he was physically at
a place where his body would be well able to
metabolize several vaccinations at one time. Three
pokes to his leg, some tears, and a consolation trip to
a local toy store and I thought the event would
quickly fade into the background of our busy lives.
Nothing could have been further from the truth.

As a mom, that day will always be a day that brings utter and complete dread to every cell in my being. On that day, I made a choice on behalf of my child that was a game changer. I will never be able to shake the sense of responsibility I feel for my choice. All I can do is continue to work for my son's healing and tell our story in the hopes that it saves another family from unwittingly going where we have been— a place I would not wish upon my worst enemy.

I want to make it clear that I am not anti-vaccines. I chose a delayed vaccination schedule for Anychild not because I am against vaccines, but because I believe there is a safer way to inoculate our children against childhood diseases. I do not intend to entertain the controversy that surrounds this issue; my point is just to tell our story.

Childhood vaccinations are necessary—of course they are and this complex and highly charged subject is not one I intend to explore in this book. If you as a reader are adverse to the mention of vaccines, please keep reading. *Our story has little to do with the vaccine issue at large.* In our case, a particular combination of routine childhood shots simply became the tipping point in a complex process that unfolded for Anychild in an acute way, shortly after these shots. We know now that if he had not had those shots, something else would have triggered the landslide awaiting us. As one neurologist said to us, "Genetics loaded the gun. The vaccinations just pulled the trigger."

What we know today is that Anychild has an immune system that does not function normally. We did not know this earlier in his life, because Anychild had seemed so healthy.

This flawed immune response, coupled with the three 'live' vaccines that were injected into his system that day, in addition to other factors that we will never be able to identify, created in his nervous system the equivalent of a 40-car pileup on a busy freeway at rush hour. This massive accident happened in silence.

Following the shots, I watched for the same physical reactions that all parents watch for. He never got a fever and he had no pain or swelling at the injection site. Nothing about Anychild gave any indication of any physical discomfort at all. I remember putting him to bed that night and feeling such a sense of relief that his shots were over and done with. Next up on our horizon was the happy march toward Kindergarten we were expecting to take in the fall. How little I knew.

As difficult as our story is, what happened as we moved beyond the fateful next morning *is something that could happen to anyone.* Anychild was afflicted with what I am calling, for now, a Shadow Syndrome. There could be no more apt name for it. As you read our tale, it may sound dramatic and over the top to you. It was.

Unfortunately, it still is, although now the over the top moments are much more tolerable because we have the comfort of a name for what ails him. It took us almost eighteen months to get to that name. In those eighteen months, as we searched for a cause for what was happening, it felt like Anychild had been abducted by someone and replaced with a lookalike child we did not know.

In the days that followed the vaccinations, a peculiar and awful thing began to happen at night. Anychild had vivid and frightening dreams that were unlike anything we had ever experienced. Although he had been a notoriously poor sleeper throughout his life, this was different. Beginning seven days after his shots, each night a few hours after falling asleep, he would wake with the kind of piercing scream you would expect if he were being impaled with an ice pick. His bedroom is a mere thirty feet from our bedroom, but by the time we could rush to his side, it seemed like it was hours too late. This did not just happen once each night. It happened every forty-five minutes to two hours until daylight came.

Night after night, we were met with the wild eyes of a child who was flailing and screaming, hitting and biting uncontrollably. His eyes were wide open, but they were clearly unrecognizing of anything around him. As he raged ceaselessly, he scratched at his face, pounded his Achilles tendons against the footboard of his bed, and banged his head against the wall. He screamed words that made no sense and the amount of brute force that came from his little body was unreal as he threw himself against an enemy we could not see.

More than once he screamed so hard, his nose began to bleed. It would take both Anydad and I to restrain him, and when we did so, the level of his terror increased exponentially. This kind of horrid scene would last for thirty to forty-five minutes and the routine went on all night long. Several times these sieges seemed unable to end on their own, and desperate to end his suffering, I struggled into an ice cold shower holding his heaving body. The water shocked him and it was like someone hit a reset switch.

These terrors would leave as quickly as they came and we were left with an exhausted 35-pound child, lying limp in our arms. In the aftermath of these horrific night terrors, Anychild was as meek as he had been wild. It broke our hearts to hear him whisper, "Please don't leave me alone," so quietly that his words were barely audible. It was as if he did not want to wake the ferocious beast that had just released him from its jaws. We began sleeping with him nestled in between us in bed, all three of us equally terrified at the thought of spending the night in any other way. He had two to five of these events every single night.

During one of them, Anydad picked him up and, in sheer terror, Anychild wriggled out of Anydad's arms and took off running to our front door and out into the cold night air. Anychild later told me that he thought his father was a skeleton chasing him. My blood ran cold as I suddenly understood why during these events he hit and bit and fought against us when we tried to hold and soothe him. When he looked at us, he saw monsters. When we reached out to hold him, he saw frightening creatures that were trying to take him away.

I understood, to my horror, that stepping back and letting him fight the darkness alone was the most compassionate thing we could do for him. I resorted to sitting in the corner of the room in a fetal position sobbing while he raged and fought things I could only imagine. When he quieted, I held and rocked him and promised him he would never be alone. The night terrors, at this same caliber, went on for many weeks. Sunset brought a sense of dread to our home that was palpable.

I consulted our pediatrician and he dryly suggested we follow the 'Chicago Sleep Study Method' and then said that he would have his nurse call later with a psychiatric referral. He didn't want to see Anychild. When I pressed for another solution, he said if it was that bad, perhaps we should bring him to the emergency room during the event.

I got off the phone and felt soiled by his indifference. He never heard from us again after that day. Because of my own background in the behavioral sciences I knew that if we brought Anychild to an emergency room, we would likely face being forced to hospitalize him. Both Anydad and I felt that his symptoms would be quickly labeled as psychiatric, when we deeply believed that they had a biological origin. For this reason, we struggled through these first long weeks without seeking medical intervention. It is a choice I have been grateful for every single day.

About two weeks into this new hellish existence, our days began to mirror our nights. Anychild began having daytime hallucinations. He often saw a green snake that was floating around the room and following him. When he would try to show it to us, it would disappear, sometimes slithering into a crevice in our rock fireplace. One particularly horrific afternoon, he saw a giant hole open up in our floor. As he stood pointing at the hole he was witnessing, he began jumping around wildly saying that bugs and spiders and snakes were crawling up into our house.

During these episodes we were unable to console him. He ran from us and could not hear anything we said. To try and hold him made things worse, so all we could do was watch him struggle though his own private hell and wait until the storm in his mind abated enough that he could once again hear us.

Anychild became acutely sensitive to sound and light. We had to buy heavy fabric and drape it across the windows of every room he spent any time in. He became exquisitely sensitive to noise, as well. If a motorcycle whizzed by us while we were driving, Anychild would scream and cover his ears. If a neighbor was running a snow blower or shop-vac, it would send him into agony.

Anychild began doing very bizarre things, like sitting upside down on the couch with his head where his bottom should be, rocking back and forth incessantly, yelling nonsensical statements over and over. There were other odd physical contortions that he would do as well, and he would sometimes hold these odd postures for hours at a time. I would pepper Anydad's workday with pictures of these contortions and we would share our confusion and exasperation at what was happening to Anychild and us.

During these early weeks, Anychild would sometimes scoot on the floor like an animal, or pound his feet against furniture for long periods of time. He was full of rage and belligerent and it became common to hear him say things like, "I hate you. I wish you were dead. You are the worst mother in the universe," etc. While screaming these things, he would run at us, hit us, kick us, and writhe around in a way that was surreal. It was almost like watching a seizure. In the aftermath, when his voice and body had quieted, he would whisper, "I'm sorry I said that. I love you."

His speech changed, and his cognitive growth at school completely stopped. He began stuttering profusely and his inability to get his words out resulted in instant rage. Anychild would no longer recite the alphabet, and he stared blankly at us when we tried to help him sound out the words.

He became a sudden behavior problem at his preschool. He was intrusive and unable to sit still. One day during circle time he stood up and started chanting the word 'no' incessantly. He had to be removed from the room. Prior to this there were no discipline problems with Anychild, as he was innately shy and did not want any group attention. Picturing him chanting repetitively in front of his peers was excruciating, because we knew this was not Anychild.

He rocked and writhed and insulted us verbally and began displaying self-harm. When agitated, he plucked out his eyebrows and eyelashes. This was alarming and took the level of agony one notch higher. Anychild became highly ritualized in his life; everything had to occur in the same sequence, in the same way, at the same time each day, or he went into a rage of epic proportions.

He experienced extreme separation anxiety. He quite literally could not be alone in our home, at all. Not for one minute. If I had to make a trip to the bathroom, I had to call Anydad in as a replacement.

If I was home alone with him, I could use the bathroom that was near the room he was in, as long as the door was open and I was talking to him the whole time that he could not see me. If one of us was in the same room with him, but he could not see us (for example, if we were standing behind him), he needed continual verbal feedback from us so that he knew where we were in time and space.

It seemed odd to us that he had no anxiety at all about being left at school. In hindsight, I now understand that this was because he was never alone in this setting. Group settings were actually soothing to him. There are other things, many dozens of other things, some small, some idiosyncratic, some downright scary and horrible, that he/we endured during the initial six-week period that followed that early morning trip to the pediatrician.

CHOICES

It was at this time we began doing Internet searches on topics like 'Early Onset Bipolar Disorder,' 'Childhood Schizophrenia,' 'Oppositional Defiant Disorder,' 'Intermittent Explosive Disorder' and on and on and on. Any parent who has been in this place knows the agony that comes when daring to put a name to what you are enduring. Although my background is in psychology, childhood mental illness is not my forte, and I had no specific insight to draw from clinically.

I, in fact, could not summon the strength to look squarely in the direction of mental illness. It was Anydad who first typed in the words 'Early Onset Bipolar' and began to acknowledge this possibility. We were shattered as we read down the symptom lists of these serious and devastating mental illnesses, because he seemed to fit somewhere among them. It was early March and we were beginning to acknowledge that what was happening to Anychild did not seem to be a passing phase. He was not improving and our entire lives were beginning to fall into disarray.

It was at this time that it suddenly dawned on me that all of this had begun within one week of his vaccinations. It took almost a month and a half for this realization to come because we were not looking for a smoking gun . . . we were just trying to survive what was happening.

In hindsight, I think the severity of what had happened so abruptly was so shocking that we did not realize how deep and how fast we had fallen. The first days we thought of things as 'isolated incidents.' As days gave way to weeks, we thought Anychild was just in a 'bad phase.' We thought maybe it could be incoming molars, an ear infection, etc. These hopeful scenarios kept us in a state of suspended disbelief as we hovered over what was happening, trying to place it within the context of something that made sense to us.

What was happening in our world did, of course, cause us to reach toward medicine for an answer. The few places we contacted gave us quick, hard answers that made us recoil. As things progressed and got worse for Anychild, we knew that a trip to the doctor was going to land us smack dab in the middle of a psychiatric diagnosis.

And indeed, the varied medical professionals we visited simply referred us to psychiatric counseling and mentioned a variety of drugs that might assist with his hallucinatory, delusional and bizarre behaviors. Each time we described the sudden onset of Anychild's behaviors and how they followed his vaccinations, they all looked at us the way one looks at a child stating they want to be President of the United States someday. As we spoke, we could see our words reflected in the glass of their non-seeing eyes.

I may not have found any allies in the medical community early on, but I sure as hell found an enemy to focus on. Something had happened to Anychild when three needles were plunged into his right thigh. Anychild did not suddenly become mentally ill.

Something was attacking his body and brain and I was going to root it out, hunt it down and destroy it. I remember saying to Anydad, "If we end up with a psychological diagnosis and him being on medication, so be it. But we can't start there." That was the battle cry as we headed toward the enemy. Anydad was with me, but it was I who led the charge. I may not have looked like a warrior on the outside, but I had become one and I may as well have had a 5000-man army standing behind me.

Today, I know I am not unique in this fierceness. Now that I have interacted with hundreds of other Anyparents, I know this is what we do. Unlike some other Anymoms, I was lucky, because I was not alone in the fight. I had an Anyhusband standing next to me—bearing witness to every horrid moment of Anychild's journey. His role was no less important than mine, but it was very different.

Anyhusband was effusive and unwavering in his support. He continued to work, provide, stabilize, and gave me his full trust and faith in my ability to heal Anychild. He never questioned, doubted, or secondguessed one thing I did. He never complained as he watched me, Anywife, move through periods of bitterness and isolation. Had he spoken up and wanted a voice in the battle plan, I would never have tolerated it. I had no want of another opinion. When I took Anychild to the doctor for his shots, I started the battle. It was I who would fight the war.

When the realization of the vaccination link to our situation occurred, I was finally able to mobilize a game plan. I started doing research on autism, particularly the form of autism that occurred with sudden onset and in close proximity to a vaccination. The information on this topic was plentiful, the controversy immense and the detractors of the autism/vaccination link were many. No matter, there were aspects to the stories that other families told that were hauntingly similar to what we had experienced with Anychild. That being said, vaccinations are not the topic of this book. I am not anti-vaccination. I am pro-truth. Anychild's unique truth was that a series of childhood vaccinations had been his tipping point for something terrible—what that 'terrible' was, we did not yet know.

I knew Anychild did not have autism. He was five-years-old and had been developmentally normal the length of his life. But I conjectured that whatever might be occurring to infants that have a sudden onset of autism or autism-like symptoms after a vaccine, could be happening in some form in the nervous system of Anychild. I began learning about the biomedical approach to curing autism, and reading stories from mothers who had 'recovered' their children from the precipice of this difficult diagnosis, helping their children to function at the highest level possible. It was not a perfect fit, but it was all I had.

I dove into the research, spending every spare hour I had investigating this pathway. I was astonished at what I learned. I was even more astonished by these mothers and what they had been through and what they had accomplished for their children. I took bits and pieces of each story with me into every day, and became part of an army of mothers who were recovering their children from the shadows of something often unnamed.

Even though our journey was different from theirs, I was not alone. There were thousands upon thousands of Anymoms in front of me. The way was in no way paved, but these women had been cutting and clearing a path for a long time. I wept at the sense of sisterhood that filled me. Even though Anychild did not have autism, I knew that the fire that raged within him had to be sparked from the same flame.

I created a game plan based on what I read. By the end of March we had begun a Gluten Free/Casein Free Diet (GF/CF) and added a few dietary supplements, N-Acetyl Cysteine, Fish Oil, and L-theanine. I began keeping a journal and the first entry after these changes reflected a few improvements: "Began GF/CF diet and things have been a little better. He hit me in the face this morning—is still very aggressive, but we went bowling in the PM and he had fun and could tolerate some noise. Overall, good night. No night terror."

We had begun to have occasional nights that did not include night terrors. This was monumental and the first time since the ordeal had begun that we had a break from these horrid nighttime events. Although he did continue to have persistent night terrors, they decreased in number after this. Things were far from normal, but with these diet changes and the addition of brain supporting supplements, we began seeing immediate positive results. He was a long way from okay, but the one symptom that disappeared completely was the daytime hallucinations. He was having no abnormal visual or auditory experiences. This was wonderful. Of all the symptoms, the daytime hallucinations were the most harrowing and frightening. The fact that they stopped gave us tremendous hope.

As the weeks wore on and my research continued, I quickly learned that chiropractors were my new best friends. Many of them clearly understood what was occurring in our world and were compassionate and helpful. They spoke the language. I could say the word vaccine and they did not look away. They knew and encouraged the GF/CF diet.

It was amazing to me that I saw so many other families like us in their waiting rooms. I remember thinking as I sat in one of these waiting rooms that perhaps when one falls down the rabbit hole of a sudden onset neuro-psychiatric event with their child, the rabbit hole splits into two chutes, one that sends you to a psychiatrist and the other that sends you to a chiropractor. If there were other chutes, I did not see them and no one pointed them out.

I brought Anychild to a chiropractic neurologist who asked that we get a battery of blood tests done on him that would help us to pinpoint what was happening in his nervous system. We did and the results were staggering. He had a severe inflammatory response and it appeared to be related to, if not triggered by, wheat. He also had very strong cross-reactions to milk, casein (which is a milk protein), soy, oats and nuts. There was a lot to talk about, but there was one set of results that the doctor circled and said had extra relevance, 'Transglutaminase –IgG and IgA.'

I stared at the words and numbers that meant nothing to me. Anychild had acutely high levels of many of these, even though his body had not had any wheat or gluten for many months. The chiropractor explained that these markers show a very specific type of gluten-mediated inflammatory immune response. He went on to say that these same markers are the ones they very often find in the brain of schizophrenics upon autopsy. I heard his words in slow motion and then my mind went completely numb. I looked away, tuning out the words that followed, turning as far away from this reality as I possibly could. What I heard him saying was that Anychild had schizophrenia.

Even though my head was turned, the doctor continued to speak to me at close range. When I continued to look away, he repeated my first name to make me turn back to him. His use of my name was like a smelling salt to 'wake me up' and make me pay attention to what he was saying. When I finally was able to listen again, he spoke with an authority and a firmness I still remember.

"Anymom, in the 1800s they called this 'Bread Madness.' It is sudden onset psychosis that is brought on by wheat, or what we today call Celiac Disease. Anychild has Celiac Disease and it has resulted in symptoms that mimic schizophrenia and mental illness." I was stunned, gobsmacked, completely awestruck— then jubilant and a thousand other positive emotions all at once. I had just been given a piece of information that could help us to make sense of the last few months of our lives.

With this bit of information revealed, I got very emotional. The tears came and came, not the gentle kind, but the kind that make your shoulders heave and your head throb. After months of tracking something wild in the wilderness, I had just caught some rare, elusive animal that the rest of the world didn't think was real. I held that blood test in my hands and stared at it for a long time. I had been a warrior for Anychild before that day, but in many ways I was armed with only my own conjectures. Now I had something to hold onto. That piece of paper was like a shield that I held up for protection.

This doctor said that Anychild had Celiac Disease. I was not sure that it was a definitive diagnosis, but at least we now had a name to put on what was happening.

This turned out to be just one in a series of startling discoveries we made over the next year, but we had won the first battle. We had a diagnosis. This blood test was then followed up with a specific genetic test (done through Kimball Laboratories) that confirmed what the chiropractor had found in Anychild's blood work. He indeed, possessed an HLA allele, which is one of the genes that causes Celiac. When I learned more about Epigenetics and how stressors in our lives and our bodies can switch genes on and off, it made sense that Anychild became 'suddenly Celiac' after his vaccinations.

With the GF/CF diet, Anychild continued to improve. I hoped against hope that everything we had experienced was due to Celiac Disease and waited for life to continue to normalize. He was far from healed, but we were light years away from the horrid two months we had endured in the beginning. He continued to have daily rages and behavior issues. He continued to have a multitude of sensory issues to light, sound and texture. The night terrors were still occurring, but had decreased in their number and severity.

We settled into this reality as a family. And by the way, our Anyfamily is a family of five. We have two older Anychildren. They were eighteen and twenty when their little brother and both of their parents all but disappeared from their world. They both still lived at home, yet almost from the beginning of this ordeal, they began to spend more and more time anywhere else.

The daytime raging and the incessant night terrors were taking their toll. Our older Anychildren could not sleep, they could not study, and they could not watch TV or relax in our home. They could not have their friends over because what was happening in our home was uncontrollable, unpredictable, and quite frankly, embarrassing. Whatever had carried our Anychild off those many months ago had also effectively chased our older Anychildren out of the house.

Years later when the haze over our lives cleared a bit, they were able to share with me how abandoned and forgotten they felt. I can't even write those words without tears streaming down my face, because the reality of having emotionally abandoned my older children is so hard to face. Although powerless to change the past, I will always regret it.

To the outside world, our daily life would have looked like a really, really awful episode of 'Super Nanny.' Many well-meaning friends and relatives gently implied that perhaps what Anychild needed was a 'good swat on the butt.' My ears always heard this as, "You are a bad parent creating a bad child."

For Anydad and me, every single part of our world was held hostage by what was happening with Anychild. The majority of our time and attention each day went to doing whatever we could to keep Anychild from going off the rails. Anychild never slept for more than a few hours at a time, and I was the Anyparent who stayed up with him all hours of the night. Sleep deprived, depressed, and overwhelmed, I stopped making lunches for our older Anychildren, quit asking about their days, and did not have the energy to check on what time they were coming home at night.

Anydad was beside himself and felt lost and hopeless. He immersed himself in his work, and when he was home he would spend endless hours working fervently to keep Anychild busy and consoled. In many ways, the night shift with Anychild belonged to me, and the day shift was Anydad's. Parenting Anychild was exhausting, and this hard truth filled us with both shame and dread. The stress it put on our marriage was immense. We never had people over to our house and most friendships faded away or at the very least became a shell of what they once were.

We brought Anychild to occupational therapy where he was tested and assessed for a variety of things. We were told that he had 'Severe Sensory Processing Disorder' or SPD. SPD is a neurological disorder that results from the brain's inability to integrate information received from the body's five sensory systems responsible for detecting sights, sounds, smell, tastes, temperatures, and the position and movements of the body. The brain normally forms a combined picture of this information in order for the body to make sense of its surroundings and react to them appropriately. The ongoing relationship between brain functioning and behavior is called sensory integration. Anychild's sensory integration system was faltering; this is why lights and sounds he couldn't control were unbearable to him.

He also displayed a particular manifestation of this disorder called 'Sensory Seeking.' This means that he seeks out sensation and activity *because it is soothing to his nervous system*. We certainly could not argue with this diagnosis. Anychild thrived with activity. In fact, after we changed to the GF/CF diet, he rarely acted out in public or during social events, nor did he become belligerent and violent, as he often still did at home.

We began to keep detailed logs of his behaviors. It became astonishingly clear that Anychild's rages, violence and belligerence always occurred under the same circumstances. As soon as things got quiet, whenever there was not a high level of stimulation, he would suddenly turn into a different child. This dynamic left our friends and family puzzled when we described the hell we were living in. They did not see what we saw because it always occurred either at home, or when we were driving in the car with him.

Often, I would pick him up from school to hear his teacher say that he had a great day. I buckled him into his car seat and closed his door and before I could get my driver's side door open, he would be screaming. Transition times became our nemesis. I cannot tell you how horrifying and deflating it is to look forward to seeing your beloved child after his school day, just to have the reunion deteriorate into an ugly, rage-filled event within minutes of pick up. His school was about three miles from our house. The things that occurred in that three mile ride were astonishing.

He beat against the car windows, kicked them with his feet, threw anything that he could get his hands on, and said the most horrific things. He spit food across the car, upended his car seat, and raged endlessly for a reason that did not exist. What this does to you as a parent is hard to describe: anger, shame, exasperation and disbelief. These are the things that we experienced on a daily basis on the drive home from almost any activity.

As we learned more about Sensory Processing Disorder, we were able to see these regular outbursts as a necessary release valve to his struggling nervous system. A neurologist explained that throughout his day, Anychild collected a certain amount of 'static' in his nervous system. The static came from periods of decreased stimulation that occurred in his day. If he had to sit and read quietly for fifteen minutes at school, this created static for him. Being physically still was almost painful. The 'static' hypothesis helped us to understand why Anychild sometimes complained that he could hear bees buzzing in his ears and head.

We knew that Anychild wanted to be good. He wanted to fit in with his peers and he wanted his teachers to like him. And although you could not tell by looking at him, he worked incredibly hard all day to hold himself together. Other than an occasional impulsive act (usually silly) that got him in trouble, Anychild fared well during this time.

As time went on and we learned to help him modulate these sensory issues, it often looked like nothing more than his being very fidgety and unable to sit still. When it became more severe, he reverted to quietly pulling on his eyebrows and eyelashes to self-medicate. If faced with a lack of stimuli, Anychild would sometimes still rage, get belligerent and display behaviors that we would rather he not, but with the education we had been given about SPD, we made our home a safe place for him to do this.

Learning about SPD helped us understand and tolerate the rages that were part and parcel to what Anychild was going through. The rages were often repetitive in nature, meaning he would do something like kick the couch repeatedly, or repeat a word again and again. If it went on for more than a few minutes, it became like a record getting stuck. When this happened, we learned that to break the cycle, we needed to shock his system. We slammed a book on the counter, rang a bell, blew a whistle, etc. Doing any of these things was like hitting a reset button. The repetitive behavior would stop and he would then be able to self-regulate.

Living this way was hard, but we constantly reminded ourselves that his struggles were due to biological reasons. These awful rages are not very different from a diabetic who begins to shake and sweat when they have a sugar drop. Shocking Anychild by slamming a book on the counter was really no different than grabbing a syringe full of insulin and plunging it into a thigh.

Despite what the outside world might have thought, we were not bad parents and we did not have a bad child. Anychild's nervous system was fickle. He and many in his generation have circuits that behave differently than we expect. That altered circuitry is invisible to the eye, but for Anychild, it's often in the driver's seat of his world. It's our job as Anyparents to keep the road as straight and predictable as we can, and to keep the road clear of debris when a neurological monster takes the wheel. When Anychild went off the rails, he was no more than a passenger in a vehicle that moved in a way that horrified him as much as it did those around him.

During this time period, I was in utter isolation with my struggles. Sure, I had friends who listened and family to lean toward for support, but I often felt minimized by their responses and defensive of the quick fix solutions they offered. Anydad and I resorted to videotaping what was going on in our home as a way to validate to others what our reality was.

The response to this ran the gamut from flippant responses about Anychild needing a good spanking, to those who couldn't watch the videos because it was too hard to see what Anychild went through on a daily basis. The physicians that we showed these recordings to rarely batted an eye. They simply tried to usher us off to various forms of therapy, both for Anychild and our family as a whole.

I did have one precious, immutable, ever present Anyfriend who, during the height of our ordeal, I called every single morning. I put on the speakerphone and she listened to the 45-minute rampage that occurred when Anychild woke up. He hit and kicked and bit me. He would have to be physically restrained during violent rages. If I let go of him to save myself, he would become even more hysterical. No amount of soothing talk or patience could reach him. The storm just had to run its course. My girlfriend listened each morning faithfully on the other end of the phone. She was horrified and later told me that she would sob and be absolutely rocked by what she was listening to, but that she knew I needed her to bear witness to my hell.

My isolation as a mother changed one day in October of 2012. We attended a birthday party for one of Anychild's classmates. I watched this child cover her eyes in horror as her birthday candles were lit. She began ranting and flailing her arms. She screamed as the tones of 'Happy Birthday' trailed off into silence and kids and parents looked around with confusion.Unless I was grossly mistaken, I had just seen another Anychild!

I could not help myself as I approached the mother and asked if her Anychild had begun having abrupt and uncontrollable behavior changes that seemed to come from nowhere. The look on her face told me everything I needed to know. A few days later found this mother and I comparing notes and feeling astonished at the way our paths had paralleled. We have become confidants since then, talking often since that first meeting, and I don't know where I would be today without her. I remember the first time she asked if I had ever heard of PANDAS. At that moment the word meant nothing more to me than the cute little bamboo-eating creatures that one sees on TV.

PANDAS is the acronym for 'Pediatric Autoimmune Neuro-psychiatric Disorder Associated with Streptococcus A.' (It is also called Rheumatic Fever of the Brain and Autoimmune Encephalitis.) Regardless of the moniker, I had not heard of any of the things she mentioned. I went home and looked up PANDAS online, but I did not delve deeply. It sounded horrible and complicated. I was not yet ready to entertain this black and white bear, because I was still pinning my hopes on Celiac Disease and Sensory Processing Disorder.

I further diverged away from thoughts of PANDAS by hypothesizing that Anychild had never had strep throat. Other than an ear infection and one virus, he had not had any significant physical illness. Anychild had never even had a fever (ever), and I had always taken comfort in what an astonishingly robust immune system he seemed to have. So I dismissed the notion of PANDAS and continued on in our GF/CF/SPD world, though by this time, the GF/CF diet had expanded to include all foods that presumably caused inflammation. This meant no gluten, dairy, soy, beans, nuts, nitrates, chemicals or additives of any kind.

Armed with little more than this diet and our careful watch, we spent our days walking gingerly through the minefield of Anychild's world. And it did not seem to matter how carefully we stepped. Many times each day we heard the 'click' of a landmine as his nervous system was triggered and the torrent of rage emerged. When something 'triggered' him, of course we saw the big outward upsets, but we also began to gauge the size of the internal explosions, as well, by some subtle indicators.

The most telling of these were Anychild's eyes. When he was triggered and raging, the pupils of his eyes became enormous. The terror stricken look on his face would fade when the rage stopped, but his pupils stayed enormous for many hours afterwards. His Autonomic Nervous System was failing at doing its job and his body was in a state of heightened responsiveness long after the stimulus was gone.

Sometimes after he had calmed, he and I would play the 'eyeball game' and see who could look into Anydad's flashlight the longest without blinking. The 'flashlight' was a phone-camera flash and we were documenting the difference between my pupils and Anychild's. Because my nervous system was normal, my pupils would constrict to pinpoint when flooded with a bright light. Anychild's were large, like black balloons against the cool blue horizon of his eyes, and stayed this way for hours on end.

During this time period, he constantly moved from one state to another: rage-filled, depressed, hyperactive, obsessed with one object and phobic of another. It was not an ideal way to live. It was exhausting for sure, but it was doable, although some days just barely.

*Of Note: More attention is being given to the link between sudden onset Neuro-Psychiatirc Disorders and vaccinations. The following article was published in the peer reviewed open-access journal **Frontiers in Psychiatry**. This article, titled: _Temporal Association of Certain Neuro-psychiatric Disorders Following Vaccinations of Children and Adolescents: A Pilot Control Study_. This study provides preliminary epidemiological evidence that the onset of some pediatric neuro-psychiatric disorders, including OCD and some tic disorders may be temporally related to prior vaccinations.

Authors: Douglas L. Leslie, The Dept. Of Public Health Sciences, Penn State University, Pennsylvania State University College of Medicine, Robert A. Kobre, Brian J. Richmand, Selin Aktan Guloksuz, and James F. Leckman, Yale Child Study Center, and the Yale University School of Medicine.

On December 8, 2017 the Advisory Commission on Childhood Vaccines was scheduled to discuss the addition of **PANDAS, PANS, and PITANDS** to their list of acknowledged vaccine injuries in children. This book was published prior to the outcome of this hearing. You can check the outcome at: https://www.hrsa.gov/advisorycommittees/childhoodv accines/. Better yet, contact your senators and members of congress and become a voice for our Anychildren.

DESCENT

Enter February, 2013. One year had passed. We awoke to the howling sound of Anychild in the throes of a night terror. He had stopped having them, so we had moved him to his own twin bed that was in our bedroom. Even though the space between he and I was no more than four feet, by the time I heard the screams, I may as well have been four miles away. I

pulled him into my arms as he screamed words of
hatred into my face with all his might. He buried his
foot deep in the softest part of my stomach and
kicked, knocking the wind out of me. And just like
the air in my lungs, he was gone.

An immediate sickening familiarity washed over
me as I backed away from my flailing child who was
now screaming, "Do it! Do it! Do it!" over and over.
Just like before, his eyes were wide open, but they
were unseeing. It was not until I splashed icy cold
water in his face that the firestorm stopped. We got
him quiet and laid him down between us and he went
back to sleep.

It was 1:00 a.m. and my mind was racing. I was
sure he had eaten gluten. I scoured my mind for what
the culprit could be. Feeling certain it was nothing he
ingested on my watch, I mentally condemned his
teachers at school, Anydad, and a litany of other
innocents who might have forsaken Anychild with
food he could not tolerate.

Our world with Anychild was so tightly
controlled, it was unbelievable. I spent hours each
week scouring grocery stores and reading labels. I
drove hours to attend Gluten-free expos, I ordered
foods that arrived in cases of dry ice, with shipping
fees that tripled the cost of anything he could eat.
The GF/CF diet was my only lifeline to Anychild and
I clung to it exactly as one would if they were lost at

sea. I did not yet know it, but that lifeline was about to give way.

Over the next three weeks we made a rapid and dismal descent back to all we had just escaped from. I think it might have been worse than our initial descent into the underworld, because this time we were not naive. As we tumbled hopelessly down the pit that seemed to have no end, there were mile markers that we recognized: night terrors, extreme violence, hallucinations and frantic hyperactivity.

This time there was a noticeable uptick in his rigid thinking patterns. He was completely unyielding in his demands, which were often unreasonable and even nonsensical. "Make the sun stop shining," he bellowed for hours one morning— yes, for hours. He became obsessive about foods and how they were prepared and placed on his plate. He often became consumed with one food and would eat it exclusively for weeks on end.

He had to have his vitamins lined up in a certain way *before* he saw them. If he saw them prior to their being placed in a perfect line, it did no good to place them the way he wanted. By then it was too late, and they had been ruined. He raged and reacted and controlled and demanded from the moment he woke up until the hour we laid him down at night.

He began needing to collect things, a desperate and horrible kind of need that was like watching an addict look for a fix. At one point it was dollar bills. He needed to stack and straighten them and if one of his dollar bills would not lay perfectly flat he would go into a rage and shred it into pieces. He became phobic of bathing and would not let us wash his hair. There was a time when he would not succumb to bathing, period. Many, many days would go by and other than outings to a local swimming pool, he could not tolerate any water on his body or head. We coped with this by keeping his hair cut short to the scalp and spoke to no one of our predicament.

As all of this occurred, I felt like we were surrounded by giant neon signs that had fingers pointing downward with the words, "THIS WAY TO HELL" written in bold red letters above them. We were devastated. I was inconsolable and utterly defeated. I made an appointment with our family doctor and went on anti-depressants. We would get through the mornings and deliver Anychild to school where he did surprisingly well. I would hold myself together in public and absolutely fall apart any moment I had the chance. Anychild was tumbling back into the dark night and because I was holding tight to him, I was going right along with him.

Once again, we visited a doctor, a new neurologist, and upon hearing the word 'vaccine,' the only finding she noted was that his tonsils were large. She did not want to run any tests, but would see us back again in six months. Scratch that. She would see us back never.

After that, I was done with our local Anydocs. Thankfully our local Familydoc knew me well enough to listen and support us medically in the minimal ways he could, but he did not understand what was happening to Anychild and could offer no cure or answers.

With my friend's urging (remember birthday party Mom?), I got a referral to an out-of-state doctor. I called and made an appointment with the same physician who had been helpful with her child, whose journey had been so similar to Anychild's. I did not know what we were hoping to find, but we had nowhere else to turn. So the appointment was made and a few weeks later found us on a plane heading far away from home.

This doctor is one of the few PANDAS-literate clinicians in the country. He spent a full hour with us and listened to our tale with keen interest. He commended us for everything we had accomplished thus far, and he apologized for the shame that had been heaped upon us by physicians who did not believe our story. When I told him this had happened to Anychild after his vaccinations, he looked away and said that his Anywife lives with my same grief because of something similar that happened to their Anychild. He did not say so, but I am guessing this is why he is a PANDAS clinician.

At the end of our hour, he said he wanted to run a variety of blood, stool, saliva, and urine tests on Anychild. He predicted two things: that Anychild would have strep and that he would be homozygous for something else called MTHFR. We headed out of his office and I remember feeling deflated. I did not think that strep bacteria could be present in a child as robustly physically healthy as Anychild. As for MTHFR, I thought it sounded just shy of a very dirty word to me, and gave it no more thought.

The days passed and the results of Anychild's tests arrived in the mail. There were fourteen pages of lab results. As I focused on the numbers, I literally had to sit down. This could not possibly be Anychild's blood work. What I was seeing made my head spin.

His strep titers were through the roof—his blood was teaming with this horrible germ! But it was not just Strep A that had made a home within Anychild. Mycoplasma Pneumonia, HHV-6 and Epstein Barr had all set up house in his bloodstream, as well. Every one of these intruders had been found in levels many hundreds of times higher than what is considered normal.

Anychild, who had always seemed so healthy, was not healthy at all. Anychild was sick. Very sick. How could a child who never had a fever in his six years of life, be so sick? I could not yet comprehend it.

He was also positive for that almost dirty word, MTHFR. The PANDAS doctor informed us that this meant, among other things, that Anychild should never have received three live vaccines at one time.

Perhaps most shocking and telling of all was that his throat culture also came back positive for Strep A. *The strep that was there had not even been hiding. It was in the first place to look, but no one had bothered to consider it.* His stool analysis showed his GI tract was swimming in Strep A, as well as a variety of other nasty microbes that should not be there. Other tests revealed that many of his neurotransmitters that assist in regulating mood, sleep, and the Autonomic Nervous System were scarce to nonexistent.

I was in shock. I called our Familydoc and had throat swabs for strep A done on every one of us in our household. (Some people can be 'carriers' and test positive for strep when they are asymptomatic.) I also had all the same blood work that had been run on Anychild, run on me. I did this thinking that the results might be similar, hoping that maybe everyone's blood work looked like this if put under a microscope.

I was wrong. Of course, I was wrong. None of us showed positive or abnormal results for anything at all. All of the strep swabs were negative, and I was left to sit with the unbelievable thought that perhaps a simple strep throat infection had been what had caused Anychild's world to career into hell.

Because it was not just strep that was swimming through Anychild's system, he quickly moved from a PANDAS (Strep A) diagnosis to PANS (Pediatric Acute Onset Neuro-psychiatric Syndrome.) This simply meant that Anychild's immune system was reacting in the wrong manner not only to strep, but to several other viruses and/or bacterium, as well.

"Your child has PANS." How stunning it was to hear the doctor say those words. I felt strangely neutral at first; then I was euphoric because I finally had a culprit to blame. I had not realized, though, what an elusive culprit it was and that the PANS diagnosis would not put an end to the other pieces of the puzzle—the Celiac Disease and the Sensory Processing Disorder (SPD). I was overjoyed to know that this illness was treatable, but I was grossly naïve about what a controversial hotbed we had just stepped into.

Today, I view the last few years of our descent into the underworld like this: PANS drove the bus to hell; Celiac Disease and SPD were simply passengers that came along because they could. Bacteria and viruses can enter and exit the bus at any given time; a motley crew of drifters is common with many PANS kids. For Anychild, vaccines have a seat on the bus, too, as well as other genetic, environmental and biological factors. Though I will never know for sure because of the long period between onset and diagnosis, my mother's heart believes it was strep that took the wheel that day when the light in our Anychild suddenly went dark.

The following explanation of PANDAS comes from one of the first PANS-literate doctors who treated Anychild:

"PANDAS is a relatively new explanation for a very old disease—the spread of strep or rheumatic fever to the brain. The terms are about fifteen-years-old and established by Dr. Susan Swedo of the National Institutes of Mental Health (NIH/NIMH) in the mid-1990s.

PANDAS describes a group of children who seemingly overnight develop symptoms of OCD (Obsessive Compulsive Disorder), involuntary movements (tics), mood disturbances and other serious health problems following an infection with GABHS or strep bacteria, as in a simple strep throat, or scarlet fever. With PANDAS, the strep bacteria is able to cross the blood/brain barrier, resulting in neuro-behavioral symptoms.

Other symptoms may include the sudden appearance of eating disorders, behavioral regression, anxiety, sleep problems, hyperactivity, learning disorders, behavioral problems or bedwetting.

These children have an immune system that is unable to get rid of the strep, even with antibiotics. They may be genetically prone or have some kind of problem with their immune function. Through a complex mechanism, their bodies end up producing antibodies that cross the blood/brain barrier and attack the child's own brain, producing an autoimmune reaction in the basal ganglia, thought to be responsible for the child's symptoms.

As a newly recognized illness, there is much controversy within the medical community around whether or not PANDAS exists, how to diagnose it and how to treat it. It requires a new way of thinking about these childhood disorders and not all providers have been open to doing this yet. NIH held the first ever conference on PANDAS just this past summer, and a mere twenty physicians and researchers from around the country and world attended. Thus, most physicians and pediatricians have not yet heard of PANDAS, and insurance companies are lax in covering treatments.

At the same time there is a growing evidence-based library of peer-reviewed medical literature and success stories of children diagnosed with PANDAS who are treated appropriately. PANDAS was in the news over a dozen times in 2010. There are a number of networks and blogs and information banks that share information about PANDAS and a movement to educate physicians to "Think PANDAS" when a child presents with sudden onset of neuro-psychiatric or tic disorders.

Many parents of children with PANDAS tell a similar story. Their child was fine until a specific date and then everything changed. Usually, at least in retrospect, they can identify a strep infection within months prior to symptom onset. Often they end up going through a series of doctors and health providers before finding someone who 'Thinks PANDAS' and actually diagnoses their child. Many others figure it out themselves by spending endless hours researching online and finally finding someone to do the testing.

Treating PANDAS is complex and unique to each child's presentation, health and length of PANDAS symptoms. With active strep most children require antibiotics, and we do whatever we can to minimize their impact on the GI tract.

Many PANDAS children already have digestive problems such as Celiac Disease or Dysbiosis (imbalance of bacteria in the gut) resulting in nutritional deficiencies or other inflammatory disorders which we try to correct in the process as well. The standard of care for treating PANDAS may include additional medications as well as IVIG, or intravenous immunoglobulin."

*NOTE: Pediatric Autoimmune Neuro-psychiatric Disorders are an evolving and mercurial group of illnesses. From this point forward, the acronym PANS will be used to represent all forms of Pediatric Autoimmune Encephalitis, as well as PANDAS and something called PITANDS (Pediatric Infection-Triggered Autoimmune Neuro-psychiatric Disorders).

We are forever grateful for this doctor and diagnosis. When you can name your enemy, you can fight it. We don't know for sure how long Anychild had PANS prior to diagnosis. He was a temperamental and easily flustered child from birth, but never to the point that it made us think that there was actually something wrong with Anychild. Within days of his vaccines, it was clear and undeniable that there was something horrible happening to Anychild. In retrospect, we believe that the vaccines acted as a catalyst to his PANS—the vaccines did not cause PANS—but essentially acted like gasoline that was dropped on a fire that had been smoldering for a while. He may have cycled through some mild flares before this, but nothing severe enough had happened to warrant further attention.

Anychild had PANS. This caused us to do a huge U-turn in our lives and took us into a world full of new challenges. Once diagnosed, under the tutelage of our PANS doctor, Anychild began swallowing more doses of horrid antibiotics than you can imagine. Three times a day for months on end we begged, pleaded, and sometimes forced these concoctions down his throat. He took anti-yeast medicine daily and anti-virals twice a day. He took anti-inflammatories and immune modulators. I became expert at hiding a variety of powdered medicines in everything from applesauce to puddings made from strange things like kudzu and chia.

Why kudzu and chia? Because Anychild was gluten free, dairy free, soy free, and nut free and remained this way for over two years. He quit asking for ice cream, but never gave up asking for Goldfish Crackers. Watching Anychild long for the simple foods he once loved and regularly saw his classmates devouring was heartbreaking. Yet, Anychild was a trooper. When forced to give up his beloved Kraft Macaroni and Cheese, he surrendered to eating its paltry replacement without complaint.

Our house often had the unusual odor that came with a PANS delicacy called 'Bone Broth.' This pungent broth made from slow cooking chicken or beef bones for days in spring water with a dash of apple cider vinegar, helped to replenish the enzymes that the antibiotics in his system robbed from him. I made huge batches of it to freeze so that it could be added to every savory food Anychild ate. It was routine to spend $400 dollars every single week on groceries as I worked to feed Anychild clean, organic, gluten free, dairy free, soy free, nut free foods that we believed would eventually help bring his system back to homeostasis.

Along the way, women I had never met became some of my closest friends. They lived across the country and like me, spent much of their lives on a Facebook feed for mothers of PANS children. (I know—a Facebook feed as a savior sounds ludicrous. Trust me, it is not.) This 'Secret Facebook Group' was like an underground village I dropped into every day, where I could be naked about our journey and ask gut wrenching questions of other mothers who also lived in the underworld of PANS. Others cannot see these closed Facebook pages, and in order to be allowed on the page you must have a child with a PANDAS or PANS diagnosis. Being accepted onto the page requires almost an Act of Congress, because PANS parents can really only afford to be real with other PANS parents. The admins of these pages are incredibly thorough when they check out the Anyparents who apply for membership. I know, it sounds like a secret society.

That's because IT IS.

An outsider reading some of the posts on a PANS page would likely peg the children *and* their Anyparents as crazy. Ironic that it is the one place Anyparents can go to stay sane. Words can never reflect how grateful we are for the cyber web of Anyparents we have met and interacted with on these pages.

These pages and groups are mostly comprised of Anymothers—and these Anymoms are not just supporting and educating one another. They are also hard at work learning to put PANS in a cage. The Anyfathers have their place, too, but from what I have seen, that place is usually somewhere behind the Anymothers. An army of Anymothers, who have the ear and the knowledge of a handful of physicians who are willing to listen to them, is quietly mobilizing.

The wealth of information these women hold about this disorder is astonishing. The things that have happened to some PANS families across the country (think Child Protective Services and involuntary psychiatric holds befalling children who just need antibiotics) make it a pretty close knit group, despite the distance and lack of physical contact shared between members.

You see, without a doctor to listen and to diagnose, it is hard to have a voice. These secret Facebook groups allow Anyparents to speak their fears out loud, ask questions, and often for the very first time, begin to see how astonishingly similar our Anychildren often are. I shudder to think of the thousands of families who fall into the abyss of a sudden neuro-psychiatric change in their child and get dropped by their physician straight down chute number one into psychiatry. If these families were to hear the word PANDAS, like me in the past, they would think of nothing more than a cute black and white bear. I ache for them, and I ache for their children. PANS/ PANDAS is not a catchall diagnosis, but it is not rare.

Today, I believe without doubt that it has close cousins in Autism, Asperger's, ADHD, and a myriad of other disorders that have all exploded in frequency among our children. Brain inflammation, gastro-intestinal imbalances and a leaky blood/brain barrier are probably the culprits more often than we know in many of the ills that are befalling our Anychildren. Yes, I have my theories, but the hard evidence is for the scientists to figure out.

For now, I will simply say that I believe there is a torrent of Shadow Syndromes afflicting our children in massive numbers, disorders that are inflammation-based and neuro-psychiatric in nature. They carry the shadow of many other syndromes that never quite fit, and they cast their own shadows that leave families with NO light because a modern medical system is failing them and their children.

VENT

Despite the fact that PANS is being studied by the National Institutes of Health and has garnered attention from top physicians at Harvard, Yale and Stanford Universities, the traditional medical community continues to cast doubt toward the Anyfamilies of this world who travel long distances and pay out-of-pocket for medical care that they cannot find in their hometowns. In August of 2016, the University of Arizona opened the world's first Children's Postinfectious Autoimmune Encephalopothy Center of Excellence. Families from all over the world are included on their waiting list.

Yet here in Anytown, USA, PANS still seems to be a dirty word to the majority of doctors we have had the misfortune to need over the past years. In our hometown, when we say that Anychild has been diagnosed with PANS, many clinicians say they have never heard of it. If they have heard of it, they often say that the clinical data does not support it and treat us like we are parents who do not want to admit that Anychild is mentally ill or incorrigible.

This makes the Anyparents of this world want to sit these clinicians down and tell them our stories, detail-by-sordid-detail, although many of us have done just that and it has gotten us nowhere. Anyfamilies endure being shamed, shut up, and scoffed at by doctors and countless other individuals who think for some reason there is a kickback to having a sick child.

Do these people truly think that Anyfamilies want to live this way? If indeed, our Anychildren were *just* mentally ill and could take a pill to quell their symptoms, do they honestly believe that we would withhold a medicine that might release our Anychildren and us from this hell? Do they care enough to learn that historically PANS children decompensate tremendously on psychotropic drugs and that it can take many months to recover them from these pharmacological insults to their already failing nervous systems? Do they know that some Anychildren, once forced onto psychotropic medications, never recover from the effects?

To the Anydocs who treat Anyfamilies as if PANS is a convenient excuse that we use for whatever it is you think we are trying to avoid—I speak directly to you here.

What do you believe are the hidden perks to having a child with PANS? Would it be the shame? The isolation? The despair? The sense of failure that we feel as parents? Is it the exasperation we feel at watching an invisible enemy pummel our child neurologically, when we can do absolutely nothing about it?

Or maybe you think the draw is the special way we learn to move through the world, continually scanning the horizon for other children that could be ill so that we can steer our children quickly off to the other end of the playground? Is it the way we become over reactive and somewhat obsessive and compulsive ourselves as we man the gate against the stealth enemy of strep always lurking somewhere just beyond our line of vision? What is it that makes you believe we wantonly coaxed PANS through the front door of our lives?

Admittedly, we do get the added bonus of our children being the odd man out when social events like sleepovers come around. A PANS child often does best in a regimented and known environment—and as much as our Anychildren want to enjoy sleepovers and other spontaneous hallmarks of childhood, the unpredictability of these types of events is often too much to risk. Do you surmise that there is some secret feel good that comes from keeping our Anychildren out of these activities?

Or perhaps the draw is from all of the awkward conversations and sideways glances we get to enjoy from neighbors, teachers, other parents, and even some of our own family members?

Or maybe you think we enjoy the perk of forced attendance at the parental online education, Google-search, home schooling/correspondence program that so many PANS parents enroll in during the wee hours of the morning when we cannot sleep— searching prompted by the latest symptom set our Anychildren are displaying. Anyparents also get to enjoy full membership in those secret Facebook groups that are all the rage.

Most Anyparents get to enjoy the cognitive deficits related to stress and sleep deprivation and watch it affect all aspects of their lives negatively, every single day. But perhaps this is a small price to pay for the many obscure info bites that our brains are able to hang on to, like what a Single Nucleus Peptide is and why a mutation called MTHFR can be an important factor for our Anychildren. Most Anyparents understand what mitochondria do and why they matter. We grasp the concept of leaky gut syndrome and understand at a very deep level how a breakdown in the blood/brain barrier is what can make or break our Anychildren on any given day.

And the vocabulary expansion that comes with PANS is impressive. It often includes words like dysbioisis, methylation and Obligate anaerobes. Anyparents learn to fear a bacterial infection called C. diff, that Saccharomyces Boulardi lyo is the best probiotic to chase down the heavy doses of Azithromycin with, and we learn that there is a secret grief that comes with the realization that no matter how good things might get in the future, we will never be able to get the past back and that what our Anychildren have lost, we will never be able to replace.

Yes, all you doubting, shaming, scorning Anydocs: As you can see, PANS is a hoot, a place us Anyparents arrive at purely for our entertainment and to receive extra special attention.

SLIP

For several months after Anychild's PANS diagnosis, he steadily improved. As strep was eradicated from his system, we saw so many positive changes it made us believe that perhaps the cure for Anychild's PANS was going to be a one-and-done massive dose of antibiotics. Our optimism did not hold up against the reality of PANS.

Despite following every direction we were given, and pumping Anychild full of antibiotics religiously, the descent came again, out of nowhere. Like a group of mountain climbers rappelling down a sheer face, we lost our footing. Our PANS doctor acted quickly and treated aggressively. Anychild was put on three different antibiotics at once.

The harness of medications held, and our descent bounced to a halt, but I was devastated. With all we had been doing to prevent a relapse—how did yet another microbe manage to push through Anychild's blood/brain barrier? I became hyper-vigilant and overprotective of Anychild. Knowing we lived on the edge, that every day brought with it a hundred different things that could loosen the ground beneath us, was taking its toll. I worried incessantly about Anychild, wary of just about everything the outside world held.

I began to research environmental toxins, pesticides, airborne forms of mold, anything and everything that I thought might be able to send Anychild back into the autoimmune abyss. It was an exhausting mental state to hold, but it's hard to relax when you look down and you cannot see the bottom. My mother's fight or flight system was in overdrive. Yet the more I learned, the more empowered I became. And the more I learned, the more I realized that we were lucky.

Our story was mild compared to many. Although our daily life with Anychild was like an unpredictable ride on a neurological rollercoaster, most of his symptoms were occurring behind closed doors. With our tightly managed routines and regimented way of living, we were managing to live with PANS largely contained within the confines of our own home. Anychild attended school, played on sporting teams, and functioned exceedingly well despite the symptoms we worked against daily.

Some of the families we have gotten to know have lived through things I cannot fathom. The losses are often too many to count: marriages, family relationships and financial stability fall away. Families routinely give everything they have to the fight against this elusive enemy.

Severe Obsessive Compulsive Disorder (OCD) is one of the primary manifestations of PANS. It is not uncommon to hear of children who suddenly become germ-phobic and begin washing their hands so frequently that their skin peels and bleeds. And the compulsions that they are struck with can be so strange and debilitating that they are kicked out of schools and their parents are turned into Child Protective Services. The OCD alone can create enough chaos to completely upend the functional lives of entire family units. On the secret Facebook page, sometimes Anyparents will post heart wrenching videos of their Anychildren lost in the ritualized world of an OCD attack. It is harrowing to see just how far down the OCD rabbit hole PANS can take Anychildren.

Anychild, at his onset, did have acute OCD, but when we began the GF/CF diet, it quelled those flames considerably. We never reached the full OCD crescendo that we know is possible with PANS. Our path has not been an easy one, but with a few key choices made near his onset, we tamed Anychild's brain inflammation early. We believe these early interventions have made all the difference in the world.

HOLDING THE LINE

As we picked our way along the precipice of another PANS remission, it became more and more difficult to continually seek all of Anychild's medical care out of area, so we began looking for a local pediatrician who would see Anychild for the antibiotic prescriptions he so frequently required. I saw two different local doctors and brought with me to our initial visit my huge binder of information on Anychild's history. Their responses were lukewarm at best and they both made it clear they would not be prescribing antibiotics for a phantom illness. One of the doctors, when hearing my report of Anychild's erratic sleep pattern and total inability to sleep for more than a few hours at a time, suggested that we do a sleep study. I jumped at the offer; more information was always a good thing.

When the results came back they showed that Anychild's oxygenation saturation levels while sleeping would dip as low as 82% and his pulse rate would race up to 214 beats per minute. Anychild had sleep apnea. This created an actual response in a local pediatrician, and Anychild was referred for a tonsillectomy. This was something that research had shown could be a game changer for some PANS children.

After this, we made the informed decision to have Anychild's tonsils and adenoids removed. Although we had no choice but to have the surgery in our PANS-illiterate hometown, we were successful at finding a surgeon who said he would consult with our PANS doctor. Our PANS doctor carefully explained Anychild's history to the surgeon and requested that Anychild's tonsils be cultured after they were removed so that we could get a better snapshot of some of the microbes that were likely some of the biggest culprits in our PANS battle. The surgeon verbally agreed to this plan.

Anychild tolerated the surgery well, and at the post-surgery follow up appointment with the local surgeon, I was anxious to hear the culture results. The surgeon had admittedly been noncommittal when Anychild's PANS diagnosis had been touched upon in our presurgery visit, but I had not noted actual discord toward it, so I was unprepared for what occurred.

The appointment drew to a close and the surgeon had failed to bring up the topic of the tonsil culture, so I asked about the results. Honest to God, he actually smiled as he said to me, in the most sarcastic tone imaginable: "Oh, the culture that your 'PANS' doctor ordered? I decided not to run it. We only do cultures on really sick kids here. You know like transplant kids...." With that bombshell statement, he shut the chart and excused himself from the room. Our window into looking at what lurked in Anychild's system had just slammed closed and there was not a damn thing I could do about it. Once again we were sucker-punched by a medical system that is vested in shunning Anyfamilies that do not fit into a convenient medical model.

Although Anychild had no complications to speak of from the tonsillectomy, our PANS doctor had warned us that the surgery was likely to stir things up, and that his symptoms might get worse before they got better. As expected, a few weeks after the tonsillectomy, Anychild fell into a serious flare. With antibiotics and antivirals onboard from our out-of-area doctors (the local surgeon was helpful with none of this) the flare was kept in check.

About three weeks after this surgery, it appeared that something had shifted within Anychild, and for the first time in a long time, we had a semblance of a normal life with our son. For six weeks, we had nary so much as a blip on the PANS radar. Unbeknownst to me, we were about to blindly head straight into another flare.

Monday morning, October 7th, rolled around and Anychild and I arrived to the pediatric dentist for his routine checkup. It is not an exaggeration to say that this dentist was visibly moved when he saw the proud, brave and beaming Anychild sitting up tall in the dental chair, opening wide for his exam. This dentist had witnessed our horrific descent into hell in the previous year and had experienced Anychild's rages and anxiety during his dental exams. Anychild was like a different child on this day. He was so proud of himself: he spit, swished, and swallowed on command. I took a picture of Anychild during his exam and sent it to Anydad. As a family, we were all beaming at our small victory.

I did not realize that we had just opened the gate. As the dental hygienist had picked away at Anychild's teeth, unseen microbes had lined up like ants heading for a picnic basket. Because Anychild's blood/brain barrier is compromised, a system that should operate like a wall instead operates like a revolving door. That revolving door swung around lazily as it delivered those microbes straight to his brain. By October 14th it was clear we had a big problem. The night terrors, rages, and rigid behaviors came back and once again, the plunge into the abyss began.

I knew we were on our way back down, but there was no way I was going to let Anychild hit rock bottom. On the secret Facebook page that was my lifeline, I had been reading about a doctor on the other side of the country from us who had dedicated the last several years of his practice to unraveling the mystery of PANS. He was one of the few clinicians I had heard of who was willing to work with families at a distance and over the phone. I know consulting with a physician thousands of miles away sounds like a dysfunctional way to utilize medical care, but for PANS families, it is sometimes the only way. Although we had no plans to discontinue working with our original PANS doctor, we felt that adding a second PANS-literate physician to Anychild's care was a good idea. The more knowledge the better.

Farawaydoc was in high demand as there are so very many children afflicted with this disorder who do not live within proximity to any PANS-literate doctors. Anychild was descending quickly; I had nothing to lose. I Googled his name and up popped his phone number. I dialed. It was a Sunday night. I fully intended to leave a message. To my utter astonishment, the Farawaydoc himself answered the phone.

I stammered out a bit of our story and he very kindly assured me that he would have his secretary set up a phone consultation with us the next day. True to his word, I got a phone call from that secretary the next morning and we were on the books for a phone appointment later that day. I faxed every record I had to him along with my meticulous timeline of where Anychild had been over the preceding eighteen months.

Unlike the doctors who grimaced when I told them I had a detailed history of events to share with them, Farawaydoc actually sounded impressed with my careful documentation. I was shocked that by the time we had our phone consultation that afternoon, he had ingested every bit of information on Anychild I had sent him. He wasted no time. He ordered a battery of tests that were so extensive, the lab tech demanded that we split the draw into two separate visits because of the amount of blood they needed (eighteen vials). After it took four adults to hold Anychild down for the needle stick, she agreed to finish the order with just one visit. Call it compassion in action.

Farawaydoc was a man on a mission. He tested for all of the known culprits which showed up as expected in Anychild's bloodstream, but he also tested for a plethora of other things that would help us begin to better understand the firestorm that had ravaged Anychild's system. Among the many telltale signs of infection that showed up in his lab work, there were also high levels of anti-adrenal antibodies. Although we were given no definitive answer as to what this might mean, it was clear Anychild's system had the ability to attack its own tissues mistakenly.

We were getting a clearer picture of that forty-car pileup that happened in Anychild's nervous system the day he got the vaccinations. Among other things unknown until then, his body had turned against his adrenal gland.

There was not much we could do about this situation other than observe. Farawaydoc kindly agreed to call a pediatric endocrinologist in our area to explain our plight and ask that Anychild be followed for observation. The endocrinologist agreed to take Anychild. This was a huge step for us—a local doctor who heard the word PANS spoken out loud and was still willing to see Anychild. My hackles went down. A little.

That referral proved to be a very positive experience. That endocrinologist was the first local pediatric doctor to give any legitimacy to PANS. She followed Anychild's unusual adrenal issues for several years, and although she never treated him for his PANS directly, she never questioned that his diagnosis was correct or legitimate. Her simple willingness to walk with us on our journey and hold an attitude of open minded compassion was a gift I will always remember.

After the results of all of these labs were metabolized, the game plan for Anychild was carefully laid out before us. He would continue on his GF/CF diet and he would begin a litany of antibiotics and antivirals to combat what his dental appointment had stirred up. He remained on these high dose medicines for many, many months.

Because Anychild was now grappling with several autoimmune issues (Celiac, PANS and high anti-adrenal antibodies), in addition to the antibiotics and antivirals that he was taking, his PANS doctor also prescribed an additional transdermal medication called LDN (Low Dose Naltrexone) that had been shown to have an immune modulating effect.

With our game plan in place, we set off into the future . . . armed only with a handful of medicines and a strict diet. It was slow going, but over the next few months, we began the precarious ascent out of hell. It was gradual but consistent and pretty soon, little victories began adding up. Anychild was laughing. He was playing. He was simply living his life. Truly, only Anydad and I knew what it had taken to get there. As a trio, we were battered and bruised, but nevertheless, we patched up the broken places and kept moving forward.

Anychild did incredibly well after this course of treatment. In fact, life became astonishingly normal at our house. Anychild began to sleep in his own bed—we moved a sleeper sofa into the sitting room that was just outside our bedroom door and this became Anychild's nighttime perch.

He was happy and free of all traces of neuro-psychiatric symptoms. He was performing at grade level in school, playing sports and socializing just like every other child his age. Anychild was off all medications other than the transdermal cream that helped modulate his immune system; it and the GF diet were the only remnants of the PANS hell that we had been living in. It was an easy load to bear—we had even added dairy and all other foods besides gluten back into his diet, with no ill effects for Anychild.

It was a carefree time for us. For month upon blissful month, life was really good. Anychild had a few blips on the radar, but nothing that some Advil and TLC did not get us through. For a very long while, there was nary a symptom of PANS proper. I convinced myself that perhaps with the GF diet and the continued use of immune supportive agents, Anychild's system had finally begun to modulate itself.

SNEAK ATTACK

Then Spring of 2015 rolled around and it was time for Anychild's biannual dental cleaning. Because his link between flares and dental work was well established, we had begun using prophylactic antibiotics prior to Anychild's dental exams. Using this approach had proven effective, and Anychild had experienced minimal reactions to his last few cleanings. I had no reason to expect anything different with this one.

Our appointment day arrived and found Anychild
sprawled in the dental chair complying happily with
the dental hygienist's urgings to allow 'Mr. Thirsty'
(her suction tool) to inhale all of the 'sugar bugs' she
was finding as she shined and polished his teeth.
When we left the office that day he took a quick look
through the prize bin and decided on his usual: a
plastic paratrooper figure with a flimsy parachute
neatly folded on its back. As was typical, two steps
into the parking lot, Anychild launched his newly
acquired paratrooper high into the sky. The chute
never opened and the figure careened straight back
to earth with a thud. At that moment I had no idea
how prophetic this moment would later seem.

Four days later was a Sunday morning, my usual
grocery-shopping day. As was typical, I left the house
at 7:00 a.m. to begin my trek to the three different
grocery stores I frequented. I had practically earned
a degree in gluten free living and keeping Anychild
interested in GF fare was a full time job I took quite
seriously. Combing the grocery aisles for a new food
he either could or would eat became a near obsession,
and these Sunday morning trips were one of the few
'predictable' things I had managed to create in my life
as an Anymom.

I was only at store number two when my phone
chimed with a text from Anydad. "When will you be
home? Anychild says he doesn't feel good." This was
unusual but not alarming. Anychild still awoke most

mornings with a stomachache and joint pain, so this day's complaint did not immediately raise any red flags. I finished my shopping and headed home.

I got home and Anychild seemed quiet but not acutely ill. He had a play date scheduled with a friend for 11:00 and the first thing that he said to me was, "Mom, I can't have my play date." It was a statement, not a question. This got my attention. Anychild NEVER let a play date slip away.

I sat down with him on the couch and asked what he felt like. He could not really say. His head hurt a little and his tummy hurt a little, but there was no specific area of his body that seemed to hold his malaise. I felt his head and it seemed a little warm, so I put a digital thermometer under his tongue. I was very surprised to see it come back at 100.2. Anychild's body had been resolutely unwilling to allow a fever for the length of his young life. He had actually experienced his very first fever only a few months before this, and it had heralded what we hoped was a normalizing immune response.

There were no other symptoms, but a fever is a fever, so we settled in for a quiet day. Day ticked into night and Anychild remained unusually quiet and calm. His fever stayed steady at 101. Despite the lack of bells and whistles, I was nervous. I did not trust this calm place at all. I slept next to Anychild that night, not because he wanted me to, but because I needed to. My instinct sensed danger. The night passed without a peep from Anychild.

The next morning his fever was up to 102. An early morning phone call from a family member who Anychild had visited a few days earlier had just notified me that they had Influenza. I immediately suspected that this virus was the culprit to Anychild's fever and got him in to see Familydoc that morning.

Familydoc looked in all the regular places: nose, ears, throat, and did not see anything glaring anywhere. He came back in the room to perform a rapid strep swab. Anychild was, by Anychild's standards, as compliant as he could be, as Familydoc rammed the Q-tip far back into his throat. Five minutes later the nurse breezed into the room and announced we had a positive strep swab. This statement was routine to her, but I felt like the bottom had just dropped out of our world. As I sat and waited for Familydoc to return with what I knew would be the obligatory antibiotic prescription, my mind reeled.

Strep was in Anychild's body again. Good God! Since his initial PANS diagnosis, he had not yet suffered a 'recurrence' of strep, so I wasn't sure exactly what this could mean. Had the gates to hell swung open quietly and we were to ready ourselves for the onslaught of PANS symptoms that were brewing? Or was Anychild's body finally able to defend itself against strep in the correct way? The fact that his body had responded with a fever made me hopeful that perhaps Anychild's system was doing just what it should.

As Familydoc wrote the prescription for Amoxicillin, it was business as usual for him. Familydoc is wonderful and was at that time our only support locally for general medical care for Anychild. Familydoc was open to the PANS diagnosis, but had a minimal understanding of its complexity. He had a healthy respect for all that Anychild had been through, but still prescribed only the standard seven-day course of Amoxicillin in response to a positive throat culture. I asked for an extended prescription of antibiotics, fearful of what the strep might do once it had made its home inside Anychild.

He was kind but resolute, saying seven days was standard and would do Anychild just fine. He was an ally I could not afford to lose, so I did not argue. He smiled warmly and tussled Anychild's hair as he assured him he would be good as new in a few days. He clearly had no sense of urgency as he pulled the script off the pad and handed it to me, verbalizing standard care instructions.

He had been compassionate throughout our journey with Anychild, but he knew about PANS only what he had read in the short article I had brought him a few years prior. He was not connecting the dots in his head like I was. Anychild had enjoyed many virtually normal months, but with strep alive in his system again, we could be facing the same hell we had so recently escaped from. Even though fear was screaming inside me, I had no choice but to take the prescription, give it to Anychild and to trust.

This fingers crossed approach was terrifying, but it was all we had. We had months ago quit following up with the out-of-state doctors to whom we were so grateful. Financially, we could not afford the high non-insurance covered fee for a non-urgent phone consultation, so Familydoc had been managing Anychild's healthy period, and it had thus far been inconsequential.

So just as we were facing the stark reality that strep had snuck in through the back door, we were also facing the fact that we had no PANS-specific medical resources to consult with in order to find our way.

As we drove home from Familydoc that day, the reality that Anychild had strep throat sat shotgun. The fact that it had been many months since we had seen our out of area PANS doctor was looming like a dark cloud. We had Familydoc, but he was not a pediatrician, nor did he have ties to any PANS providers he could refer us to. I vacillated between panic and the desire to trust our prescription for Amoxicillin and allow Anychild's immune system to do what it was meant to.

By the time we returned home I had settled on following Familydoc's orders to give the Amoxicillin as directed and to keep Anychild quiet and well hydrated. We hunkered down, gave Advil for his fever and kept his antibiotic dosing precise. It was Monday. I was hoping for a return to school by Wednesday.

When I look back at this time period, I can clearly see that we were just like the little plastic paratrooper figure Anychild had pulled out of the prize bin at our dental appointment the week before. The amoxicillin was the very first tug we were making on the rip cord designed to slow our free fall. We did not yet know that the chute was not going to open.

The next few days were very quiet ones. Anychild still had no real symptoms other than a slight headache and feeling dizzy. His fever, however, was consistent and high. He peaked at 104.2 and it took ninety minutes for Advil to bring it down to 103. I kept in close contact with Familydoc who assured me that this was all a good thing and that Anychild's system was fighting strep just as it should. He said the antibiotics should have all noticeable traces of the bacteria well controlled within thirty-six hours.

Sure enough, thirty-six hours later Anychild did seem a little bit better. His fever was down to 99, but he was still eerily quiet and subdued. His schoolwork was piling up on our kitchen counter and before we knew it, Thursday morning had dawned and he was still feeling bad. In addition to Anychild not feeling well, during the night Anydad had begun to cough and feel achy. He was asleep in our bedroom fighting a fever of his own when Anychild woke up at 5:00am with a howl. "My legs, my legs, my legs," was his hysterical chant.

I thought he had a charlie-horse and quickly swooped in to massage his calves where he was indicating the pain was coming from. The minute I touched his legs he recoiled dramatically. His chant, "My legs," continued and he had a wild look in his eyes as he bellowed. There was a whole lot of drama going on, which immediately made me think that this was a ploy, and Anychild was trying to eke out one more day without having to go to school.

Using my best tough love voice, I demanded that he stand up. He shook his head, insisting that he couldn't. I playfully swung him off his bed and placed both of his little legs squarely on the ground below him. As I released my hands from under his arms he went down like a fallen marionette. I was flummoxed and still not sold on the severity of what was happening. Having a leg cramp was believable enough, but being wholly unable to walk? That seemed unlikely.

It did not matter how I cajoled, bribed, or demanded, Anychild was adamant that he could not walk. Not knowing what else to do, I went and got our digital thermometer and placed it under his tongue. After a week of watching the thermometer shoot up to 101 before he could even close his lips around it, I was shocked to see those digital numbers rise up oh so lazily from the 95 mark. It took a full minute for his temperature to reach 96.2.

I was certain that we must have run the batteries on this thermometer low during the week, so I quickly grabbed another one from our medicine cabinet and gingerly placed it deep into the pocket of flesh beneath Anychild's tongue. I urged him to keep his mouth tight around it and to breathe through his nose. I think my own temperature may have dropped a few degrees as I found myself peering at another thermometer that was struggling to climb above 95 degrees. This time it topped in the low 95s. I looked closely at Anychild's legs and could see that from the knees down they were slightly mottled. I touched them and they were cold.

I have been a mom for over 26-years and in that time I have taken my share of temperatures. I had never seen a temp in the 95s and whether it should have or not, it panicked me. The fact that his temperature seemed to have dropped from the 96s to the 95s in the several minutes it had taken me to find a second thermometer was unnerving, never mind the fact that Anychild could not walk!

I woke Anydad up and showed him both the thermometer reading and the mottling on Anychild's legs. As he struggled to understand my rapid fire speech, it became clear to me how sick Anydad was. Touching the back of my hand to Anydad's brow, his fever was apparent. I urged him back to bed and hit the ground running with Anychild in my arms. I wasn't sure how dangerous this low temperature was, but I knew that something was very wrong. With a final shout goodbye to Anydad, we were out the door and on the freeway in a few minutes flat. I fought against the tears that wanted to erupt from my eyes.

What the hell was happening? My worst fear with Anychild was to land in an Emergency Room and to have a physician misread Anychild's PANS symptoms and treat them in a way that could cause irreparable harm. But Anychild could not walk and his body temperature was nearly four degrees below normal. This was not something I could handle on my own. I knew my fear would ignite his, so I did my best to keep the mood light and playful. As I pulled up to the hospital valet I heard myself say the words, "We need a wheelchair. My son can't walk."

The ER staff was swift and efficient. Because of his symptom-set and low temperature, Anychild had an IV line and labs done within the hour. I carefully explained to the ER doctor that Anychild had tested positive for strep three days prior, and that he had a history of PANS. She listened attentively and allowed that it was plausible that whatever was happening was his body's errant response to strep. Her open minded response to my information made me feel hopeful. My hope was short lived, because here is where 'normal' came to a screeching halt.

FREEFALL

I share what follows not only to bring attention to the medical condition that was occurring with Anychild, but also to invite you onto the crazy train ride of having a child with PANS. What was happening to Anychild was scary and stressful, but what made the experience escalate to the most frightening few days I have spent as a mother had little to do with what was occurring medically. *Instead, it had everything to do with what was not happening regarding his care.*

When Anychild's labs came back, they showed what would be expected for a system fighting an infection, but there was one value in particular that got the ER physician's attention. Because of Anychild's inability to walk, the doctor had ordered a Creatine Phosphokinase test. CPK is an enzyme found mainly in the heart, brain and skeletal muscles. When a muscle is damaged in the body, it leads to elevated CPK levels in the blood. High levels can indicate a brain injury, a heart attack, or be a sign of myocarditis (inflammation of the heart muscle). Most importantly, high CPK levels can have a damaging effect on the kidneys. Normal levels for an adult male should be between 20-260. *Anychild's first CPK reading came back at 1600.* That earned him a quick inpatient admission to the pediatric ward, where he was placed on IV fluids and swabbed for Influenza B.

They did not re-swab him for strep, so I again reiterated that he had tested positive for it a few days earlier. I assumed they would treat him accordingly, especially since I had been explicit about his PANS history. I was mindful of wanting to be clear, but also of not wanting to overstate my case. As a PANS mom, you learn there is a fine line that gets drawn in the sand between Anymoms and uninformed Anydocs. A well-informed mother will be welcomed and respected by some, and put quickly in her place by others. The ER doctor had clearly acknowledged the fact that Anychild had a current case of strep throat and I assumed he would be treated accordingly. I was woefully wrong.

Anychild was moved out of the Emergency Room and placed inpatient on the pediatric unit. With IV fluids running, he and I began to settle in. Within a few hours, the Influenza B test came back positive and Anychild was abruptly moved to an isolation room. It was after this that we were introduced to a team of pediatric Hospitaldocs. They were doing rounds and poked and prodded and examined Anychild as a group. They discussed the plan of care amongst themselves, and once it was finalized, their spokesperson turned to me and began to speak.

This Hospitaldoc was kind and upbeat. She said that Anychild had flu-related Myositis—which is basically a breakdown of the muscle tissue due to the flu. The plan for care was minimal. He would be kept in isolation and IV fluids would be given to help avoid any kidney damage due to the elevated CPK levels in his bloodstream. I asked for affirmation that Anychild would be kept on antibiotics for his strep infection, but Hospitaldoc negated my query. I was stunned. I repeated the fact that Anychild had tested positive for strep a mere three days prior to this. I tried to keep my anxiety down, but the small verbal skirmish that unexpectedly emerged was unnerving. Hospitaldoc perused Anychild's chart but remained noncommittal. "Let's see how the rest of his labs come back and we'll go from there."

Hours later, an Anyresident walked into the room and introduced himself. Hospitaldoc had apparently passed our case to him. Before he could even finish introducing himself to me, I had moved on to the first order of business: Where were the antibiotics I knew Anychild needed? I was digging my heels into the sand, ready to go full force with my plea, when this Anyresident's next statement hit me squarely between the eyes.

"According to his labs, his ASO is negative, so he doesn't even have strep."

I was stunned. I knew what an ASO titer was. It stands for AntiStreptolysin O Titer. It was one of the smoking guns that had shown up during Anychild's initial PANS diagnosis. I felt dazed.

How could Anychild's rapid strep test be positive on Monday, yet his ASO be negative on Thursday? As a PANS mother, the word strep is often the battering ram that we end up using against the walls that go up in front of us. The word creates such heartache in our lives and gets refuted by so many we do battle with. I had used the word strep confidently to inform the hospital that my Anychild needed antibiotics. I had used the word strep because I was armed with a positive culture result from just a few days earlier. And now this Anyresident was telling me that this was not the truth, that Anychild did not have strep. I felt my cheeks grow hot with shame. I was accustomed to doctors treating me like I was an idiot because of my viewpoint on strep . . . this time, I actually felt like one.

A perfect storm was brewing. I was sitting in a hospital with Anychild, who could not walk. He had tested positive for strep three days prior to this in Familydoc's office, but there was no medical record of that visit at the hospital. I had informed the hospital that Anychild had tested positive for strep on Monday and that he suffered from a controversial Post Streptococcal disorder called PANS. This was immediately followed by the Hospitaldocs informing me that Anychild's blood work confirmed he did not have strep. My head was spinning. *Did Anychild have strep or not?*

A benign scenario to most moms was deeply troubling to me. It hit at the very heart of what I most feared—that Anychild would have strep and it would somehow go undetected and take us back into hell. For so long, Anychild's life had been a medical nightmare because he had strep and no one realized it. And after we learned this truth, we still had a plethora of uninformed Anydocs who continued to wrongly believe strep was *not* the basis for his ills. And here I was presenting Anychild to the hospital stating that he had strep, when apparently he didn't. It felt like a bad dream. I was reeling and utterly exasperated by the situation. I was terrified that strep was raging unchecked through Anychild's system and humiliated that nothing in Anychild's lab report confirmed this fear.

Once again, our world was mirroring the plastic paratrooper from the week before. The ripcord was useless against the free fall that was happening and numbness set in. I was spent at that point, incapable of understanding what was happening to Anychild. Immobilized by the confusion that this entire medical experience was creating, I simply did not know what to do.

Meanwhile, Anychild still could not walk and his CPK levels were profoundly high and getting higher. These CPK levels indicated that an active destruction process was taking place in his system. I massaged his little legs and tried to push the strep fears away. I had no alternative other than to trust that the Hospitaldocs were right and that Anychild did not have strep. I curled up next to Anychild and tried to stifle my tears.

The isolation unit was most certainly doing its job. I felt like Anychild and I were a thousand miles from anywhere. Anydad had the flu and my own Anyparents were home sick with the same thing. Our older children were both immersed in end of semester finals at college, and my best friend was away on vacation. In addition to this, Anychild was contagious and visitors were not encouraged.

Anychild was growing more anxious and demanding. He could not tolerate any extra noise in the room and had to be physically touching me at all times. His behaviors were reminiscent of how a PANS flare typically begins, but I tempered this thought with the fact that Anychild had very good reason to feel cranky and anxious. He couldn't walk and his body was hard at work at destroying his muscles. I kept my PANS fears in check and just focused on my son.

Hours passed and no one in the pediatric unit seemed particularly concerned about Anychild. Strangely enough, this was both bothersome and comforting, depending on how I looked at it.

The fact that no one bothered to check if his fever was up or down could just mean that he was a low priority case and there was nothing 'big' to worry about. This first scenario is certainly the tone that the Hospitaldocs had set when they assured me that 'benign flu-related myositis' was not a big deal. The other possible scenario, that Anychild was not receiving good care and was blatantly being overlooked haunted me, but the fact that I had told them Anychild had strep when he apparently didn't haunted me even more. It haunted me enough to keep me quiet.

So there we sat, alone together, in the isolation room. No medications administered, no discussions occurred, no real attention paid to anything involving Anychild's health. The only activity in our room happened when I carried Anychild and his IV pole to the bathroom every twenty minutes or so due to the volume of fluids running through him. He weighed sixty pounds and I weigh 110, so this was no easy task.

After quite a few hours of this, I started to feel angry. I remained quiet, but the momma bear inside of me was stirring. I was puzzled by the fact that they were not measuring his urine output. He had been admitted due to the strain that a high CPK level was putting on his kidneys. Shouldn't they be interested in what was happening to his kidneys and the fluid in/fluid out ratios?

I became aware of other menial forms of negligence. Anychild had been an inpatient for over 24-hours. During that time no one bothered to

populate his bedside tray table with the obligatory
box of tissues and plastic water pitcher that are part
and parcel of any hospital admission. As Anychild
became warmer and flushed, I asked if they would
take his temperature. The response to my query
was sluggish and disinterested. Anychild's fever
was ticking back up toward 101 and he was starting
to cough and complain of more leg pain, but no one
really cared and they were not shy about letting me
know this. My anger continued to be tempered by the
fact that I was confused and ashamed that I had told
them Anychild had strep when his blood work
contradicted this.

A variety of Hospitaldocs and Anyresidents
breezed in and out of Anychild's room like a vapor
the first day. Two or three times they popped in and
continued to assure me that 'Benign Myositis'
associated with Influenza was not a terribly unusual
occurrence. There was a veritable circus of emotion
going on inside me. I was like an amateur juggler
tossing fear, confusion, anger and shame up into the
air, while trying to remain present with Anychild,
who grew more agitated as the hours wore on. While
Anychild tossed and turned and peed, I waited
anxiously to see what the next battery of blood tests
would show.

On the last pop in of the day, a Hospitaldoc sat
down to pull up Anychild's labs online. As
Hospitaldoc waited for them to load, he said, "Let's

make a bet. I'm going to bet that his CPK levels are down to normal with that last blood draw." (Blood had been taken a few hours earlier.) This doc was being playful, but I said nothing in response. His prediction was wrong. Anychild's levels had risen from 1600 to 2400. I was horrified. Hospitaldoc was nonplussed and said only that we would redraw labs in the morning and go from there.

Momma bear was stretching her limbs inside me. I knew that strep or no strep, her hibernation was coming to a close and she was going to roar very soon. At this point, Anychild could not tolerate having me even a few feet away from him at any time. And he was starting to flinch and flex in ways that worried me.

As a PANS mom, you become hyper-vigilant to any nuance of change in your child, especially any type of physical movement that could be the start of the tics that can ignite like wildfire.

When you are scanning the horizon for a flare, a typical flinch that would not even register in your consciousness during a time of health, becomes monumental because you know that unusual movements can herald a neurological change in your child.

Although Anychild had never experienced any long term tic behaviors, during acute phases of his prior flares, he had experienced a variety of short term tics, stuttering and something that looked very similar to Restless Legs Syndrome. As Anychild wriggled and squirmed beside me, I pushed my PANS fears away. He'd been in bed for two days, his leg muscles would not hold him up, and he had a virus coursing through his veins. Of course, he was going to be fidgeting and moving around a lot. Right? I prayed this was so.

Anychild's distress was clearly ramping up. The extreme anxiety he experienced anytime I was not physically touching him was reminiscent of the prior flares we had known. I countered this notion by telling myself that he was in an acutely stressful situation, so his anxiety at this point was founded.

In the past, during severe flares, he could not tolerate Anydad or me being out of earshot or eyesight when we were at home—at all. His behavior in the hospital was mirroring this exactly.

Although his hospital room was small, if I even got out of bed to relieve my own bladder using the in-room bathroom, he needed to be able to see me. Despite my best self-talk that Anychild's anxiety was completely understandable given our situation, the truth of PANS kept nipping at my heels, reminding me that we could be at the beginning of both the tics and the crippling separation anxiety that are part and parcel of a PANS flare.

I lay next to Anychild paralyzed between two very divergent desires. The first was the need to express to a medical professional that strep was raging through Anychild and that we were careening toward a hell we knew all too well. And the second was to trust that Anychild really did not have strep and there was really nothing to worry about.

When you have a child with PANS, and you have been to places with your child that no one else in the world can even imagine—and you think you may be heading back there again, it is hard to remain level headed. I was doing my best not to overreact, but I could feel panic building and it was getting harder to keep my fears at bay.

Adding insult to injury, I had not slept more than a few hours or eaten a real meal in two days. I could feel my mind becoming numb and incapable of reason. I was at a loss for what to do.

Another day was closing on our conundrum with no clear path forward. Exasperated, we settled into a restless night of sleep. Anychild still could not walk and continued to have body aches and fever. I had no idea what might be going on in his little body, but I resigned myself to embracing the benign Flu-Related Myositis diagnosis that he had been given.

Despite my attempts at accepting the diagnosis, my dreams that night were peppered with flashbacks from our past. I could not get a handle on the growing discomfort that Anychild could have untreated strep running through his system and that we were once again ticking up the tracks of the PANS rollercoaster. What if no one but me could hear the ticking, let alone see the drop that lay ahead of us? The what-if's were creating a frantic feeling inside me. I became emotional and visibly distraught, which was not helping Anychild at all. I was his rock and I needed to keep my game face on. Try as I might, the facade was starting to crack and by the time morning arrived, fear held me firmly in its grasp.

As Anychild picked at the plate of rubbery scrambled eggs set before him, his room door opened and the nurse announced that his labs from the night before were back. I waited anxiously for her to announce that the CPK value had dropped. To my great dismay, they were almost double what they had been twelve hours before. The CPK value that should have been below 100 had gone from 1600, to 2400, to its new level of 5400. All told, his CPK levels had more than tripled in a twenty-four hour period.

I was really starting to feel afraid. Anychild had been treated like an afterthought by this staff for two days, yet his body continued to get sicker and sicker. *What if his muscles were being attacked by strep and not the flu?* I also wondered if an ASO-titer could be wrong? The possible leverage of an answer to this question pushed me to get out my cell phone and do a little bit of research on 'ASO titers.' A whole host of sites came up, but the one that caught my eye was the PANS site that is sponsored by the National Institutes of Health. I clicked on the cached link, which took me directly to the portion of their site that discusses how ASO blood tests are used in a

PANS diagnosis. I read the first sentence, blinked hard, and read it again:

"An ASO titer does not elevate until three to six weeks *after* a strep infection."

This had nothing at all to do with PANS and was general knowledge about ASO titers. An ASO titer measures PAST, not current, strep infections.

I want you to pause here for a moment and pretend that you are watching one of those cartoons where a record is playing and then the record needle is suddenly pulled violently across the moving vinyl. Yes, that screech.

Take a deep breath, close your eyes and one at time slowly stretch your arms above your head. In your mind's eye, see that exhausted, distraught momma bear who had been so quiet for so long while everyone ignored her Anychild, doing this very same thing. As this momma bear completes her stretch, see both of her eyes opening with a 'plink.'

Anychild's ASO titer was normal not because he did not have strep, but because his strep infection was five days old, not three weeks old.

At that moment it was like someone hit the washer-fluid button on the windshield wipers of my clouded mind. I clicked out of that site and onto another to double check this information. Site after site after site confirmed this same truth: A normal

ASO titer less than a week after a positive strep test means absolutely nothing.

Suddenly, the shared opinion of all of the Hospitaldocs who had breezed into our room at the time of Anychild's inpatient admission, with their airtight opinion that Anychild was experiencing nothing more than a simple case of the flu gone wrong, seemed like an egregious medical oversight. Strep is the most common pediatric diagnosis made. How in the hell does a meandering group of Hospitaldocs who heal people for a living, not know that an ASO titer only becomes positive *three to six weeks* after a case of strep throat? Why did I have to consult Google in order to learn this?

At this point I had to sincerely question the quality of medical care Anychild was receiving. It seemed that once Anychild had received a positive result on the Influenza B nasal swab, all other infections were kicked to the curb by the doctor whose care we were under. It was true that a nasal swab had confirmed that Anychild did have influenza B, but as we had learned five days prior in Familydoc's office, Anychild also had strep throat, damn it! There is just no other way to say it. This Anymom was now PISSED.

I was now certain that Anychild had strep throat and he had spent the last thirty-six hours with no antibiotics in his system at all. (As is customary with a hospital admission, all of the medications Anychild had been on at home had been discontinued in lieu of the medications the hospital was giving.) Anychild's temperature continued to rise and his CPK levels rose way off the charts. He was still unable to walk and his pain was increasing, yet not one person on his care team thought there was anything to worry about.

With this new information about the ASO titer came the huge realization that perhaps it was *strep* attacking Anychild's muscles and causing his CPK levels to rise. Knowing the unusual routes strep had taken in his system in the past, I could not help but worry that untreated strep was doing God-knows-what to not only his muscles, but perhaps to his brain as well. After all, PANS is often referred to as 'Rheumatic Fever of the Brain.'

Feeling desperate to find a medical voice that could view Anychild's current scenario through the PANS lens, I put a call in to the PANS doctor we had worked with at the height of Anychild's onset. Although he practiced in another state, his location was just a few hundred miles from us, and he was the only resource I had. I was met with the devastating news that he had moved to a different state.

Undeterred, I quickly put an email out to Farawaydoc, the East Coast doc who had many months ago been so helpful in getting Anychild onto the right medications. I hit send and crossed my fingers. I also put a frantic call in to our local Familydoc. He returned my call promptly and I began to tearfully recite the litany of events that had occurred over the past two days. I shared my distress at the refusal to treat Anychild with antibiotics. He was incensed that the Hospitaldocs had refused to give Anychild antibiotics for his strep throat and he agreed with me that the care Anychild was receiving seemed unimpressive at best.

While I engaged in this phone call, Anychild lay beside me. He was anxious and demanding and it was exceedingly difficult to even try to have a simple phone conversation due to his need for verbal reassurance. I hung up the phone with Familydoc who had agreed to call the hospital and make his own request that Anychild be placed on antibiotics. I was hopeful that this nudge from an outside physician would get the antibiotics ball rolling.

While we waited for that ball to roll, Anychild and I lay shoulder to shoulder in his bed. He was twitchy and feverish and his cheeks were starting to turn red. Did he look sicker, or was my rattled mind just seeing things? I wondered to myself if Myositis could be caused by strep rather than the flu, and decided to look this up, too. I typed these two words into the search bar 'strep' and 'myositis' and hit Go. I can only describe the next thing that moved through me as white-hot fear. As my eyes focused in on the headlines of the cropping of medical journal articles that came up, there were three little words that stood out in the opening paragraphs of every single one of them. Those three words were *"rare, often fatal."*

IMPACT

What happened next is a blur even to me. I am not sure what I was expecting to find when I Googled 'strep + Myositis,' but it sure as hell was not the word FATAL. Adrenaline coursed through my veins like wildfire. I was out of that bed and down the hallway in record time. I was done sitting in the isolation room in the back of the hospital with my not very sick Anychild who "didn't have strep."

My sprint to the nurse's desk was for naught. It is not an exaggeration to say there was not one person there, not even a unit clerk. As the minutes ticked by, it became clear that, for whatever reasons, there was actually no one there. Again the feeling that I was in a bad dream washed over me. *Could Anychild be swimming in strep bacteria, which is attacking his legs and no one here is smart enough to know this? Am I being hysterical and over-reactive?*

Since there was no one at the nurse's desk to speak with, again I called Familydoc I frantically told him what I had read about strep and Myositis and ended my torrent of words with a desperate plea that he help me to get Anychild transferred to another hospital. My trust in the hospital we were in was gone.

Familydoc is a wonderful physician, and although he admittedly did not know much about PANS, he knew a lot about me and what kind of mother I am. As our family doctor for more than twenty years, he and I had weathered plenty of health storms together and he knew I was not one to cry wolf. If I believed Anychild was in danger by remaining at that hospital, Familydoc believed it too. He reached out to the on call Hospitaldoc without any hesitation and explained that I wanted Anychild transferred to another facility.

Although theirs was a conversation I was not privy to, I do know that when this Hospitaldoc balked at Familydoc's request that Anychild be transferred, a verbal scuffle of the MD kind ensued. It was during this scuffle that Familydoc was informed that if we attempted to leave the hospital with Anychild, Child Protective Services (CPS) would be called.

My face burned hot when Familydoc relayed these words to me. Child Protective Services? My fear rose to crescendo level, but Familydoc quieted my fears by assuring me that this vein of conversation went no further and had occurred only because two doctors were disagreeing on treatment options. Apparently the discussion became more cordial after this and Hospitaldoc agreed to consult with me on a possible transfer.

I was beyond horrified that the acronym 'CPS' had now been spoken in the same sentence as

Anychild's name—and all because I was unhappy
with the medical care he had received. I had to
wonder to myself, "What parent would not be
unhappy in our situation?" When I think of CPS, I
think of children who are being abused. I think of
starving, abandoned, cigarette-burned babies. I do
not think of parents who are asking for a simple
second opinion regarding their child's medical care.
Given our experience at this hospital, I think it was
perfectly understandable why I was panicked about
the lack of concern for Anychild.

The fact that a transfer could have been denied
us is disturbing, but even more disturbing is the fact
that if the transfer had been denied, I could not have
left that hospital with Anychild to seek other
treatment. If I chose to leave on my own, Child
Protective Services would have been called.
Anychild's fate was out of my hands. I was not even
sure I had a vote in what might come next.

This was such a surreal impasse to arrive at, and
my sense of exasperation was compounded by the fact
that the reason CPS was mentioned had nothing at
all to do with suspicion of abuse.

It boiled down to the simple fact that if we had
left the hospital to seek a second opinion without the
approval of a Hospitaldoc, this would have been
considered leaving the hospital AMA (Against
Medical Advice.) An AMA pediatric discharge
routinely results in a CPS referral because doctors
are 'Mandatory Reporters' (bound by law to report

even a suspicion that a child could be in harm's way) and if a parent leaves the hospital against medical advice, a doctor's liability is high.

If anyone reading this book continues to wonder why PANS parents are hyper-vigilant about germs and illness, while at the same time they are hesitant to trot their child off to the doctor, this scenario illustrates the root cause perfectly. Having a sick PANS child in an uninformed institution is a losing situation *and as Anyparents, we never know how much we might lose.*

The thought that your child could be removed from your care is paralyzing, but it is a very real possibility in this situation. It is not unusual to end up in this place of raw vulnerability when you have a sick child—any sick child. What we experienced is far from unique and unfortunately, in the PANS community, we hear similar stories all the time. The fact that parental disagreement with medical care can elicit a 'child endangerment' stance from a physician should make any parent reading this feel afraid.

As I waited for yet another Hospitaldoc to come by, I called in reinforcements. Anydad was still home with a fever, so he couldn't assist. My next move was to send an SOS out to our older Anychildren. Studying for their college finals was going to have to wait. I needed help NOW. Anychild's need to be in physical proximity to me at all times had held me hostage at his bedside for two days, but at this point, he was going to have to accept a surrogate in the form of whichever sibling arrived first. Within thirty minutes Anyson arrived, and he assumed my spot in bed next to Anychild. A Hospitaldoc arrived shortly after this and he and I stepped into the hallway to converse.

With the echo of the CPS statement still looming in my mind, I used every bit of will that I had to remain calm. Despite this, my emotions betrayed me. I tried to form a calm, even sentence, but instead I started to cry. My voice shook with emotion and I felt more vulnerable than I ever had in my life. Without warning, the anger that had been brewing inside of me morphed into something much softer. I was totally humbled by the knowledge that this man standing in front of me held all the cards, and that all I could do was hope that he chose to play them in my favor.

Any thoughts I may have held of using the ASO titers as a battering ram against him had evaporated. I didn't need to be right. In that moment, I truly believed that if Anychild continued on without antibiotics, he would be in grave danger. I just needed him transferred and given antibiotics.

I have had a lot of stressful mom moments in the quarter of a century I have been raising kids, but I had never had one like this. At no time ever had I felt that one of my children was in danger of dying, nor had I ever before felt so un-empowered as a mother.

The way I felt, to this day, remains indescribable. My fear and vulnerability in that moment must have been palpable.

This Hospitaldoc was gentle and he was patient as I tried to compose myself to speak. The words, when they came, were but a whisper. "Can we please try to have him transferred to another hospital that is familiar with PANS?" I was terrified, and I was completely surrendered. It felt like hours passed before his response came.

He was kind, firm, and agreed to call a children's hospital in a larger city several hundred miles away. But he cautioned me not to get my hopes up. He advised me that the other hospital was not likely to accept Anychild because *he was not sick enough to require a transfer.* I accepted his statement without comment but asked if he could please tell the other hospital that Anychild had been diagnosed with PANS in 2013 and had experienced what we believed was a strep-related auto-immune Encephalopothy in 2012 *and* that he had a positive strep test three days prior to this admission.

I knew I was pushing the envelope by dictating to him what to say, but I think he knew we had reached an impasse. He assured me that he would include this information in his phone call and he strode away toward the nurse's station. I matched his pace and followed right behind. He placed the call and I stood across the hall within earshot. True to his word, he shared every bit of Anychild's history, just as I had requested. He hung up the phone and looked over at me with what can only be described as a look of both pity and compassion.

I was at my wits end and he could clearly see this. He walked over to me and put his hand on my shoulder. "They will call us back in a few minutes after their admit doctor reviews the request." His kindness should have been a comfort, but instead I felt embarrassed and unsure. What if the other hospital denied the transfer? What if I was just a hysterical mother who was overreacting? I smiled weakly and thanked him and began to pace the hallway awaiting the call that would decide our fate.

I heard the Hospitaldoc paged back to the nurse's station just a few minutes later and I knew this was it. He took the call on a phone down the hall so the conversation was out of my range. With the call ended, he headed back down the hall toward me. As I looked down the hall at him, bracing myself for his words, his body posture spoke volumes. He was holding his hands up in mock surrender as he walked. When he got close enough for me to see his face, his eyes were kind and his voice was soft as he said, "They have a bed waiting for him. We just need to check on your insurance and he will be transported there by air tonight."

As those words made their way into my awareness, it felt like a thousand pound weight was lifted off my shoulders. Knowing we were heading to a children's hospital that had a working knowledge of PANS was enough to make me feel like I had just won the lottery. I quickly called Anydad and told him the good news. Even though he was still sick with the flu, he decided to don a mask and come down to the hospital to see us off.

Knowing that Anydad would soon be there brought another wave of emotion. If I was Anychild's rock, Anydad was mine. Just knowing he would soon be there brought a sense of comfort I had not felt in days.

When I returned to Anychild's room, Anybrother was still lying next to his brother, just as he had been when I left. He raised his eye brows at me as if to say: "What happened?" I responded by putting my arms out like airplane wings and casting my eyes westward. I smiled and gave him a self satisfied nod. Anybrother smiled back and I knew that he knew that his Anymom had just slayed her a dragon—and he was right.

As I sat down on the bed to break the news to an already anxious Anychild that he was going on an airplane ride, a nurse breezed through the door and added a small bag of medicine to his IV pole. When I saw the word that was written on the bag, I started to cry. My tears kept perfect time with the drops of Ampicillin that were now falling in a steady stream into the clear plastic tubing of Anychild's IV. It had taken almost two days and an unbelievable amount of effort to accomplish this simple treatment. To this day, I still agonize over why.

By 9:00 p.m. that night, Anychild and I were bumping down a runway in a small fixed-wing air ambulance. The pilot handed me a pair of headphones and motioned for me to put them on so that I could hear him. I complied and he warned me that it was going to be bumpy; we were heading into a storm. I let his words settle into me as I thought about the storm that Anychild had been fighting for three years now. Remembering what we were leaving made heading toward those dark clouds in the night sky a lot less ominous. Whatever storm was waiting, we would meet it, just as we always had.

A short forty minutes later found us safely on the ground at a prestigious children's hospital. We were whisked into a room and every single individual we spoke with, from the admitting physician to our team of nurses referenced Anychild's history of PANS and expressed concern over the sharp rise in CPK values that had been steadily occurring over the past two days. I relaxed, a little bit. Anychild and PANS were finally on the radar.

He remained unable to walk, but he was now on antibiotics. I snuggled into bed next to Anychild and fell into the first deep sleep I had managed in two days. The blood draw that was done the next morning, a mere twelve hours after beginning IV antibiotics, showed that Anychild's CPK levels had dropped by 1200 points. It appeared that his body was finally halting its attack upon itself.

This drastic change in his lab values post-antibiotics was impressive to say the least.

Now that things were improving, I felt brave enough to revisit the articles on strep and Myositis that I had Googled the day before, the ones that had sent me out of my mind with terror. Once I read the articles in their entirety, I could see that the fatal form of Myositis that was referenced in the online articles whose headlines had shocked me was a strep specific illness called Necrotizing Myositis. Having the time and the presence of mind to read the entire article, I could see that it presented in a much different way than Anychild's Myositis had. I was grateful Anychild had not faced that form of Myositis, but learning about it did nothing to change the fact that Anychild had received no treatment for the strep that raged through his body.

I reflected back on the two days that we had spent fighting for a simple antibiotic and I marveled at how things had played out.

The day I scanned those articles and saw the word 'fatal' in the headline, my whole world stood still. Anychild's uncommon history with strep should have warranted extra care, given his presentation. Yet he had remained untreated for nearly two days, while his Myositis continued to increase at an alarming rate. I could not help but wonder how and why our situation had gotten so needlessly complicated. To this day, I have no answers. Anychild's admittance records clearly show that the doctor was aware that Anychild had both a history of PANS and a current and active strep infection. Why a simple antibiotic was resolutely denied Anychild remains a mystery.

As we settled into the new hospital, Anychild remained on IV antibiotics. His fever disappeared and his energy level rebounded. Anydad had recovered enough from his bout of flu to drive the several hundred miles that separated us and he joined us the next day. It seemed Anychild was on the mend, but he still couldn't walk, even though his CPK levels continued to drop. He began physical therapy and we learned how to stretch and work his muscles to help hasten the healing process. After just three days on antibiotics, his CPK levels had normalized and he was discharged home with a small walker to support him while his ailing calf muscles strengthened.

The night after Anychild's discharge we stayed in a hotel near the hospital just in case. The night passed without incident and as morning dawned brightly, we decided to begin our journey home. We pointed our car toward home and I could not shake the ominous feeling that overcame me.

For the length of Anychild's illness, our hometown had been a virtual desert when it came to PANS and Anychild's local medical care had been piecemeal because of this. We had been on the PANS rollercoaster, but we had never been forced to seek emergency care. Given the recent viral/bacterial insult Anychild's body had just endured, we had no idea what his immune system might do in the near future. I was terrified that if Anychild should become acutely ill again, we could be forced to again walk into an emergency room and relive the nightmare we had just been through. This was terribly unsettling.

We still had our trusted Familydoc, but he did not have hospital privileges. The events of the last few days changed everything. We needed a PANS-literate doctor who had hospital privileges. As soon as we got home, I began my search. At that time, there were only three recognized PANS clinics in the country. We had been referred to the one closest in proximity to us, but we knew the odds of admission were not in our favor. They had a waiting list of thousands and their admission criteria were strict.

The first order of business upon returning home was to resume phone consults with Farawaydoc. He was nearly 3000 miles away, but he was all we had. It appeared that we were not the only ones leaning toward Farawaydoc. The first available appointment was several weeks out. I took it without complaint.

In typical Anychild fashion, his healing trajectory after the Myositis was lightning speed. By the time we got home, he was using the walker minimally, mainly for balance as he teetered on his tiptoes.

Putting his heels down was painful, but the more we adhered to the stretches the physical therapist had shown us, the more Anychild was able to put weight on his feet. His little calf muscles had been through hell, but the doctors had advised us that the more active he was, the faster he would heal, so we let Anychild dictate the pace, and dictate he did.

He had a soccer game the weekend after we arrived home, and he had his mind set that he was going to play. Using a walker on Wednesday and playing in a soccer game on Saturday seemed like mutually exclusive activities, but we remained open minded. Athletics had always been Anychild's saving grace. Even during his worst flares, his hand/eye coordination and agility remained untouched by his illness. Sports were the one place he was free, so if Anychild thought he could run, we decided that we would let him run.

Saturday came and sure enough, Anychild wanted to play. He went into the game for just a few minutes and was clumsy and sore, but like always, he was free. It felt like normal was coming back to our world—but I was still nervous. Anychild had been discharged from the hospital with just a few days worth of antibiotics. We were given instructions to follow up with his regular doctor upon our return home.

Of course, that was easier said than done. I worried that Anychild needed a much longer course of antibiotics than anyone local would be willing to give him, and made this plea by phone to our local Familydoc. He said that he would see Anychild the following week and that if he complained of a fever or sore throat before that to call. Having no other option, we tiptoed into the future, hoping not to wake the beast.

Less than a week later, the beast was awake and screaming. It was in the wee hours of a Sunday morning that Anychild woke from a sound sleep shrieking and raging. Sleep disturbance was almost always the first thing that signaled descent, and typically, once the night terrors arrived, Anychild unraveled fast. We had braced ourselves for the storm and it arrived right on time.

It was a Sunday and I was on my early morning trek, grocery shopping, when the slide into darkness began. When I returned home carrying my bevy of grocery bags, I walked into the house and everything seemed calm and quiet. Anychild was sitting on the couch watching TV, but Anydad was on his feet and making eye contact in a way that let me know he had something to show me. In silence he led me to our laundry room and opened up the washer. There was a colorful variety of clothes swishing to and fro in the soapy water.

I looked up at Anydad perplexed. Sunday morning chores were nothing unusual. Why did Anydad have the urgency to show me he was doing laundry? In silence he led me to Anychild's bedroom where

Anydad opened up drawer after empty drawer. I didn't understand. Anydad then explained to me that Anychild believed that his clothes were full of germs. Anychild had insisted that every clothing item that he owned needed to be washed. As Anydad's words continued, I quit listening and just put my hands over my face and began to cry. Anychild was displaying contamination fears and had become suddenly germ-phobic.

We had just fallen back down the rabbit hole and all we could do was spin in the darkness until the Fates decided how far the drop would be. I knew that Anychild needed to be on antibiotics, but it was Sunday, so our only option was an ER or urgent care. We were still so fragile from our last experience that we did not want to risk wandering back into a mainstream medical setting, so we opted instead to call Familydoc on Monday morning.

It was astonishing how quickly the beast of PANS took away Anychild. Any parent of a PANS child will agree that it is as if someone walked through your front door and carried away the child you know, while you stood there helpless and unable to stop it. And to make it even worse, the rest of the world often remains blissfully ignorant of the abduction process. On that day only Anydad and I knew what was happening. We braced ourselves for what we knew was coming.

That night Anychild slept between Anydad and me. My hopes that this close proximity to us would keep the night terrors at bay were short lived. Anychild was plagued by nightmare upon nightmare all night long. I had thought the terrors came only when he was dreaming, but in the predawn hours of this very long night, I learned this was not true. Needing to use the bathroom, I silently slipped out of bed. Anychild had been sound asleep beside me— or so I thought. The minute I stood upright, I heard his frantic whisper, "Don't leave me, Mommy."

I explained that I just needed to use the bathroom, but what he said next stopped me in my tracks. "Don't leave me. If you do, they'll take me away and leave a boy made of wax who looks just like me . . . and you won't even know I'm gone." I knew from his voice that Anychild was wide awake and lucid. This was not a dream. This was a paranoid delusion. I verbally assured him that I would never leave him, and slipped back into bed next to him. I gathered him up in my arms and held him, weeping silently as I waited for the dawn to come, though I knew that despite the morning light, our world had just grown dark.

We kept Anychild home from school that day, and were able to get in to Familydoc later that morning. He swabbed Anychild for strep, and even though it came back negative, he agreed to prescribe one more ten-day course of antibiotic therapy. I knew this was not enough, but at least it was a start. We began the course of antibiotics and waited for an improvement to begin.

The digging out process was never a quick one. We hunkered down, knowing the road ahead might be a long one.

Soon after this, we were able to have a phone consult with Farawaydoc. He ordered labs and changed Anychild to a more PANS-specific protocol of antibiotics, as well as an antiviral. With this new medication regime we saw swift and significant improvement in Anychild, and within a matter of days, all visual and auditory symptoms were gone. We were left with only the more basic and manageable PANS symptoms we had known in the past: extreme separation anxiety, sleep disturbance, restrictive eating, ADHD and OCD. This laundry list of symptoms, although arduous, was one we could handle.

The results of the labs that Farawaydoc had ordered arrived about four weeks after Anychild had returned home from the hospital. They showed the infections and viruses that we expected, along with a more in depth look at the CPK levels that had been so concerning in weeks prior. Farawaydoc had ordered a detailed test which broke the CPK levels of the Iso-enzymes into three different categories.

CPK-1 (also called CPK-BB) is found mostly in the brain and lungs. CPK-2 (CPK-MB) is found mostly in the heart, and CPK-3 (CPK-MM) is found mostly in skeletal muscle.

Four weeks after Anychild's hospitalization his CPK-2 (heart) and CPK 3 (skeletal muscle) were back to normal. His CPK-1, however, (brain and lungs) was an 8.0. It should have been zero. This enzyme is normally elevated only after a stroke, a seizure or some other injury to the brain. Clearly whatever had happened to Anychild during his last flare had impacted his body in ways we could only see in hindsight.

Because the acute inflammation that had led to hospitalization was over, Farawaydoc could only guess at what these high CPK-1 levels meant. He surmised that they likely reflected the attack his body had waged on his brain. It was a dismal, real world reminder of why in the weeks following his bout of strep throat, we had again returned to the no-man's land of a classic PANS flare.

If there was a silver lining to any of this, it was the fact that our 'hidden' PANS journey was no longer hidden. The fact that prior to his hospitalization, Anychild had spent many months as a perfectly 'normal' eight-year-old boy, made his sudden change in temperament evident to everyone.

His second grade teacher knew Anychild to be a good student and a compliant member of the class. After Anychild returned home from the hospital, the child she saw did not resemble the one she knew. She expressed exasperation at the level of discord Anychild was now causing in the classroom, and was astonished by this sudden change. He was rude, disruptive and weepy. He was unable to complete class assignments, and totally incapable of any independent work. He had been performing at grade level prior to this. Within weeks, his academic skills had plummeted and he was in trouble.

The elusive beast known as PANS had revealed itself in the light of day to this Anyteacher—and it turned out that she was clearly up for the battle. Anyteacher was simply awesome in the way she supported both Anychild and us. Because all this occurred during the last few weeks of the school year, she arranged a conference with the school's Educational Specialist, the vice-principal, and the teacher Anychild would have when he returned to school in the fall.

Unlike in past years, we were not going to have to tiptoe around the PANS issue, or back into it after a flare had upset the apple cart. (In the two years prior, we approached Anychild's teachers about PANS only *after* a sudden flare took him from being a normal happy student to someone unrecognizable.) Because of the last chain of events, Anyteacher knew this beast was real, and she was intent on making sure that everyone else who would work with Anychild next year would know this truth as well. The difference that this support makes to a PANS family existing alone on their island cannot be overstated.

It was not just Anyteacher who was being baptized into the reality of PANS. During this period,

Anydaughter babysat Anychild each afternoon after
he got out of school. While Anydad and I finished up
our work days, she would pick him up from school,
make him a snack and help him complete his
homework. Being our part-time nanny gave her a
bit of spending money, and it gave us the reassurance
that Anychild was in the care of someone we knew
and trusted.

Anydaughter was a young adult and a well
seasoned, long term nanny to several families, so
she had no problems managing her Anybrother. This
changed after his latest bout of strep. A few weeks
into this flare, I received an afterschool phone call
from Anydaughter. When she had gone to school to
pick him up, he was unruly and difficult. He refused
to get in her car and finally had to be physically
carried and forced into compliance. This had occurred
in front of all of the teachers, parents and other
children and Anydaughter was mortified.

Things got worse as they drove toward home.
Anychild insisted that someone had followed them
from school with the intent of harm and when they
arrived home he was too afraid to walk into the
house. He was paranoid and terrified. Upon getting
her phone call, I rushed home from work to find a
fearful Anychild and a visibly shaken Anydaughter.
As the afternoon wore on, Anychild began seeing
(imaginary) bugs on the floor and began to swat at

invisible bees that he insisted were buzzing around his head.

On this same day, Anyteacher emailed me to tell me that Anychild had refused to eat any of his lunch that day. Although he never gave her a reason for his lack of appetite, when I asked him about his uneaten lunch, he told me with wide-eyed innocence that he couldn't eat his lunch because there had been ants in his lunchbox. Anydaughter was in tears. She wanted to know what was wrong with her Anybrother.

Despite the fact that she had lived the nightmare with us, even Anydaughter had been shielded from the real horror of PANS. I gently explained to her that her brother's immune system was attacking his brain. It was causing him to have delusions and paranoia and a whole host of other symptoms. I reassured her that we just needed to stay the course with Anychild's treatment and that the inflammation would subside and her Anybrother would return.

This period marked an important transition point in our family and social system. Prior to this, Anydad and I had done a commendable job of hiding the intricacies of our PANS journey from others. Even my own Anyparents, who lived just a few miles from us and were mainstays in our daily life, had been shielded from the real down and dirty moments that PANS created in Anychild. PANS is such a wily opponent and when your child is in a full blown flare—ticking and twitching and hallucinating—the normal instinct of parents is to shield them from the world and to shield the world from them.

A PANS parent knows that this is not her child—this is an illness. But allowing those without a working knowledge of PANS to see our children during a flare is something we avoid with our whole hearts and souls. We Anyparents become masters at hiding what we can and sharing only what we must. The way Anychild's recent flare had occurred, however, broke open the truth of our world to our entire social system. It was a gift.

When Anychild was hospitalized and could not walk, this dramatic fact put him on the radar of many. Friends, neighbors and acquaintances who may have heard us vaguely mention Anychild's 'illness' in the past and who dismissed it because Anychild seemed like, well, any child, were now very concerned about his welfare. And some of this concern may have come from their own fears that what had happened to Anychild, could happen to their child, too. *How could his body attack his legs like that? Could it happen again? Is it contagious?* The well wishes were many, but the questions were even more.

Anychild is a well loved peer and a parental favorite. If we had to pick an alter ego to explain him concisely, it would probably be the cartoon character, 'Dennis the Menace.' He is an elite little athlete, the one who gets sent into the game when the score is tied and there are 30 seconds left on the clock. Yes, it makes me beam to tell you that our Anychild—he is THAT kid.

So when THAT kid spent two weeks out of school, one of them in the hospital and was then transferred to a children's hospital far away and came home using a walker, people talked. It was one of the best gifts we had ever been given because it cracked open the lid of PANdora's box, the box of shadows that we had tried to keep tightly closed to the world for the previous three years.

When we were able to explain to others that the way Anychild's body had attacked his legs was the same way it attacks his brain, the light bulb went on for almost everyone. Even those who had done their best to minimize and look away from Anychild's symptoms in the past (no one wants to talk about a child being delusional) were able to conceptualize how his wayward immune system, when hit with an incoming illness, could send its immunological warriors to the wrong battleground. His body waging its horrendous attack on his little calf muscles was the 'white crow' that allowed people to understand that in the past, Anychild's body had sent those same warriors clamoring toward his brain.

HARD LANDING

As the days after his discharge wore on and Anychild's symptoms began to subside, it appeared that Anychild had successfully navigated another PANS storm. But there was another tempest brewing, one that truly took Anydad and me by surprise.

Anychild's hospitalization brought some Anylookers to the periphery of our world. PANS families are used to the Anylookers. Anylookers are those who sit in the back row of life and cast out their judgments about PANS and all of the things that 'do not make sense' about this illness. Anylookers are unique in the fact that they have a small knowledge base paired with oversized opinions.

It was a surprise to learn that we had an Anylooker squinting through a peephole on the periphery of our world— and this Anylooker *claimed that Anychild was the victim of Medical Child Abuse.*

We did not know much about this Anylooker, but we did know that he or she was not a 'Mandatory Reporter,' meaning they were not one of Anychild's medical providers, teachers, or coaches. This was significant, because outside of home, sports and school, Anychild's interactions with others were virtually nonexistent. It was stunning that someone without any firsthand knowledge or close interaction with Anychild was pointing the 'Medical Child Abuse' finger at us, but as hard as our experience was, it could have been far worse.

Many Anyfamilies face this same dynamic from uninformed medical providers. The accusation we faced, although deeply disturbing to us, was made by someone who had very little direct insight into Anychild's world—and no medical knowledge at all. When all was said and done, it was as simple as this: We had the supreme misfortune of having an Anylooker on the outskirts of our life make a bold and very uninformed claim against us.

Regardless of how uninformed an accuser may be, when a claim of Medical Child Abuse is made against a family, things happen. And happen they did. Consequences began to swirl around us, like leaves on a blustery autumn day. Not only were we in the midst of trying to regain our familial equilibrium after all we had just experienced—now we faced the immense stressor of medical, social, and vocational scrutiny. Since both Anydad and I are licensed professionals, this careless claim infiltrated not just our personal and family lives, but our professional lives, as well.

When one is faced with a claim such as this, the only thing to do is to be transparent. To this end, we gathered together all of Anychild's medical records and corroboration of these records was obtained from his doctors. We were completely forthcoming with regards to all of his prior medical care, his recent hospitalization, and subsequent treatments.

We allowed our life as a family to be observed and scoured for any signs of discord or mal-intent, and every nook and cranny of our world was checked and cross-checked. To those who took the time to look closely at the facts, they revealed nothing more than a family that had been successfully navigating a poorly understood childhood illness and had consistently taken right action while doing so.

It took very little time to show that this preposterous claim of 'Medical Child Abuse' was unfounded, yet the fact that the phrase had been attached to our family was devastating. Never in our wildest dreams could we have imagined anyone ever suspecting us of abusing Anychild, yet there we sat, reeling from this very thing.

As the saying goes, you cannot 'un-ring a bell' and even though nothing in the real world existed to back up the claims that had been made, the alarm that was sounded continued to reverberate through our world. For all of the heartache PANS has brought forth, it has been the stain from this Anylooker that has left the darkest shadow upon us as parents.

When it comes to raising children, we all do the very best that we can. None of us are perfect, and for most parents, there are many times where we feel less than worthy of wearing the 'parent of the year' badge that we all aspire toward. Yet, for all of the mistakes we make, in general, most of us end each day knowing that we have done the best we can for our children and that tomorrow is another chance to do even better.

Openly sharing the ugly truth of this 'Medical Child Abuse' allegation with readers was a difficult decision to make, but in the end the importance of being candid about our experience became all too apparent. Through our own interactions with other PANS parents, we have learned that we are far from the only Anyfamily who has faced this horrid kind of scrutiny. I have now met and interacted with too many other Anyparents who have faced this same nightmare, and for the same reasons— *because they were advocating for medical care for their children within an uneducated system, be it medical or social.*

Uninformed claims like the one we endured, and even more serious claims such as 'Munchausen by Proxy,' are lobbed at Anyfamilies far too often. The effects of these errant abuse allegations are devastating for Anyfamilies. Perhaps most disturbing of all when considering the high number of abuse claims that PANS families seem to endure, is this fact: According to the American Academy of Pediatrics *actual medical child abuse is extremely rare.* In fact, in a clinical report published by the American Academy of Pediatrics in 2013, it was estimated that most health professionals will likely encounter only one case of Medical Child Abuse during the length of their careers.

In recent years, as more Shadow Syndromes like PANS have emerged and larger numbers of children are being diagnosed with illnesses that are not yet part of mainstream awareness, Medical Child Abuse (MCA) *investigations* have risen significantly. Yet legitimate incidents of MCA occurrences are estimated to be as low as 0.5 to 2.0 cases per 100,000 children younger than sixteen years old. (American Academy of Pediatrics Clinical Report, 2013.)

If sharing our story can help even one potential Anylooker pause and think before boldly throwing down the gavel of judgment against an Anyfamily, then sharing will have been worth it.

GETTING BACK ON OUR FEET

As the weeks wore on and the clamor of the 'Medical Child Abuse' alarm bell faded into the background of our lives, we proceeded gingerly into the future. At the time, we continued to deal, day in and day out, with the many residual symptoms Anychild was still having, while also working frantically to find a local physician who could manage Anychild appropriately, should he once again become acutely ill. We were struggling financially from the two weeks of work both Anydad and I had just missed and we were coming to terms with the stack of medical bills that were piling up on the desk. In addition to this, we, of course, continued to juggle all of the other minutiae that working parents of three children do.

Our whole world revolved around life with our children. The entire abuse debacle, although seemingly over, fractured what small semblance of normalcy we had managed to regain in the prior month. As a family, we were fragile; and as a parent, the trauma of Anychild's hospital stay and my near inability to secure the care he required had been one of the most terrifying and confusing life experiences I had ever endured. To face abuse accusations on the heels of this experience devastated me in a way that reached deeply into my core.

Mothering a child with PANS has been the most humbling, frightening, crazy-making and overwhelming thing I have ever faced. I am a confident, secure, intelligent woman. There has not been much in life that has intimidated me, but PANS on many a day has taken me to the mat. In one fell swoop, it evaporated my self-confidence as a parent, filled me with envy when I saw other families with children who got sore throats and got well, and delivered deep into my gut a sense of shame and defeat that is beyond anything I have ever known. I have had plenty of days when I have second guessed decisions I made on Anychild's behalf, but to have an Anylooker claim that we were harming Anychild was beyond my ability to comprehend. It is something that even today, years after the fact, remains a haunting and unresolved part of my life.

As an Anymom, I had been manning the ship of Anychild's medical care largely on my own. Anydad was always one hundred percent onboard, but he always deferred to me when it came to the medical decisions we made for Anychild. For this reason, the abuse claims felt deeply personal to me.

I coped with this early on by insisting that my extended family and our trusted friends sit down and painstakingly look at the facts. Intent on making Anychild's health care transparent, I acquired every single medical record, lab report, prescription, hospital record, and physician's note that I had amassed over the prior three years. I laid myself, our family, and Anychild bare, and asked those who loved Anychild most, to scrutinize every action I had either taken or had not taken on his behalf.

If there was evidence that I had harmed or neglected Anychild in any way, I insisted that they bring it forward. If there was even the slightest hint of evidence that indicated I had done anything unwarranted or questionable, I wanted it discussed openly among those I loved and trusted.

Of course, those who knew me and loved me took on this arduous task with the utmost compassion. They were overwhelmed at the amount of care Anychild had received, and the amount of painstaking attention that had been given to navigating him through the last three years. Those closest to us were shocked at how sick Anychild had been and how little they knew about what we had endured behind closed doors. Even Anydad was unprepared for the sheer amount of pure maternal drive he witnessed in the hundreds of pages of documents that lay splayed on the table before him.

At one point he asked me, "When did you have time to do all this?" His question caught me off guard, and my voice cracked with emotion as I gathered myself to give my answer. "Research is what Anymoms do at night when they can't sleep and they are worried about their Anychild."

From immunology to nutrition to genetics, I had turned over every stone I could find in my search to unearth the neurological bomb that had gone off inside Anychild in February of 2012. Prior to discovering that PANS was what ailed him, I had subscribed to newsletters spanning everything from allergies and autism, to early onset bipolar disorder. I had attended weekly support groups for Sensory Processing Disorder, invested thousands of dollars in phone consults with faraway doctors, and had read books on alternate healing modalities as varied as the GAPS diet and enzyme therapy. Especially in the early days of our ordeal, I had gathered up every scrap of information that I could, and stuffed every bit of it into the enormous red binder that Anydad was now really seeing for the first time. I was like a squirrel that had built a hidden network of tunnels that would allow me access to the things that would help Anychild.

TOEHOLD

After the frightening experience we'd had in our local hospital, coupled with the stark reality of what the Anylookers of this world are capable of, we were hesitant with every step forward after that. Navigating the stormy seas that come with PANS is harrowing. Trying to navigate them on your own, while watching your back, is even harder.

More than ever, we knew we needed to find a local doctor who could advocate for us so that we never again faced the nightmare we had just endured. The first defensive move we made toward this end was to hire a concierge physician. Concierge doctors are physicians that are retained on a private basis for general medical care and as an adjunct to any specialized medical treatments or hospitalizations their clients may face.

Because they have small numbers of clientele, they work for us and, as opposed to being seen within a large general practice, they offer a highly individualized, personal form of medical care. We gladly paid the $1600 yearly retainer and began to invest physically, emotionally, and medically into this relationship. This concierge doctor was at once both receptive and compassionate.

After carefully reviewing Anychild's medical records, he had no doubt about the legitimacy of our story. He was the human version of an insurance plan; he offered a layer of protection between Anychild and the Emergency Room. He was willing to work with Farawaydoc and quickly educated himself on the nature of PANS so that he was up to speed on what to expect as Anychild's doctor.

Under the joint care of Farawaydoc and this new concierge physician, Anychild limped into the future on a cocktail of antibiotics and antivirals. The residual effects of his flare were diminishing, yet we lived each day with bated breath because we did not know what might come next.

Even with the added layers of medical care we had in place, it was an uncomfortable time. All we had been through continued to haunt us. I became hyper-vigilant about my care and documentation with Anychild. I often brought him into our concierge doctor when I didn't really need to—because I was so afraid that perhaps I had missed something or made an erroneous mistake in caring for him. My parental self confidence was at an all time low. Daily antidepressants and a constant sense of dread became the norm as we walked a tightrope with Anychild, knowing that if strep once again found him, we had a much too fragile medical net in place to soften the fall should we once again go tumbling.

Then in mid-July I opened up my email inbox to a correspondence that would change everything for

Anychild. Farawaydoc had many months before written an extensive letter on our behalf to the Stanford PANS program. Of the few programs in the country, Stanford was the most geographically accessible to us. After Farawaydoc's referral, they contacted us and requested that all of Anychild's medical records be sent to them for review. We were warned at the time that admittance to the program was a long shot, but we held out hope.

As the months ticked by, I resolved myself to the notion that we would likely never be accepted. And then we got that mid-July email. They were requesting that Anychild be seen at their clinic later that week. They wondered if we could make it on such short notice? I read, and re-read, and read again the words in that email. Was this a joke? Was I dreaming? Anydad and I cleared our schedules and made our travel plans and by midweek we were sitting in Dr. Jennifer Frankovich's office.

It was surreal to be sitting in the same room with one of the foremost PANS researchers in the world. She was warm and inviting, but most striking of all was the outright level of compassion the entire clinic displayed. Because they watch PANS families wading day in and day out through this awful, controversial, and poorly understood illness, they make short work of ensuring that in their house, PANS families are seen, heard and validated.

As Dr. Frankovich leafed through the bright red, six-inch binder of medical documentation I had brought along, she was likely both impressed and amused by my thoroughness. She asked if it would be okay for her research assistant to take the binder and peruse its contents. I handed it over and was more aware than ever of how the contents of that binder had become like a crucible, a vessel of transformation that included both medical records and the personal narrative that was our truth.

As the research assistant left to begin her arduous task, Dr. Frankovich returned to reviewing Anychild's history with us. There was one moment in that initial meeting with Dr. Frankovich I will always remember. The question she asked was simple, a no brainer really: "How does Anychild walk when he first gets up in the morning?"

She kept her head down and her pen poised to quickly transcribe the response she was awaiting. When nothing but silence filled the room, she looked up quizzically at Anydad and me. I could see from the look on her face that she was wondering what was causing the delay in our response. She repeated the question.

I looked over at Anydad and he stared back at me—mirroring my same stunned expression. Bumper cars of colliding thoughts crashed in my head as I tried to come to grips with the only answer I had for her simple question about how Anychild walked in

the morning. I was about to tell Dr. Frankovich
something I never knew until I spoke the words.

"He doesn't."

Perhaps she thought there was a different way to
elicit a more logical response from me. She rephrased
her question. "Does he limp when he first gets out of
bed?"

Again came my stilted reply. "He doesn't walk in
the morning—at all."

This opened up an entire conversation and as I
heard the words coming out of my mouth, describing
how Anychild had long ago ceased to walk in the
mornings, I felt like I was having an out-of-body
experience. It was a bit like the TV shows you see
where someone is in a serious car accident and they
describe watching from above as paramedics remove
them from a burning car. In our case, the fact that
Anychild had not walked out of his bedroom on his
own two feet in years was the burning car.

Somehow, we never saw the flames.

Was I really explaining to this kind doctor that
Anychild had not walked after waking up in the
morning for years? For years? How in the hell did
this fact go unrecognized until today? Why had this
ridiculous oddity not been the topic of agonizing
parental debate between Anydad and I?

Suddenly, the fact that Anychild's body had
attacked his lower legs to the point of temporarily
rendering him unable to walk did not seem like such

a foreign notion. I understood in that moment that Anychild's immune system had been nibbling at his legs for years and the recent bout of Influenza and strep had just turned the immunological slow nibble into a virtual feeding frenzy. How did we miss this? My only answer is that sometimes when you are in a battle, you simply don't see the whole scene. You see what you need to see to survive.

Mornings had historically been very difficult times for Anychild. He was still frequently plagued with nightmares and slept fitfully at best. On most mornings he woke up irritable and complaining that his legs hurt, he couldn't poop, he didn't want to go to school. Some days, the list was endless.

Anydad and I had learned long ago that there were 'tools' we could use to help keep mornings from going off the rails. Top among them was carrying Anychild from his bed to the couch and giving him a good fifteen minutes to stretch and acclimate before he got on his feet. We had been doing it for so long, we forgot we were even doing it.

Despite my best efforts to stave off the emotion that had just risen in me like a tidal wave, I started to cry. Although I had no idea how this fact we just shared correlated to PANS, I was nevertheless totally blown away that we had become so adept at arranging our lives around this illness that we no longer always knew when we were arranging.

In that moment, the fact that our nearly nine-year-old child had not gotten out of bed and walked independently out of his bedroom for several years felt like a shameful confession, yet the look on Dr. Frankovich's face was anything but condemning. Her compassion was palpable as she explained that severe joint pain was common in PANS children.

The added fact that during Anychild's last acute flare all of his inflammation had settled in his calves and feet indicated that this might be the area of his body that his immune system attacked most violently. As we spoke, Anychild joined in the conversation and showed Dr. Frankovich exactly where his pain was when he tried to walk in the morning. As she examined his lower extremities, she glanced up at Anydad and I, affirming with her expression that it was all making perfect sense to her.

Anychild and his symptoms were being observed and validated by one of the foremost PANS experts in the world. In that moment, I felt like a trader on Wall Street who had just, for the first time ever, clearly and loudly heard the opening bell of the market. It had only been an echo in the background before.

After five years of navigating Anychild through a medical system that could not see him, we had finally made it to safe ground. As an Anyfamily, we had been like medical castaways, clinging to whatever we could to stay afloat. Arriving at Stanford was the equivalent of washing up on an island and realizing we could once again stand.

Since that first appointment, we have consistently met with our Stanford team every six to eight weeks. They have continued to be a port in the storm for us and have offered us the most compassionate, comprehensive, and astute medical care imaginable. They have been advocates for our Anyfamily in ways I could not have expected.

Between the Anydocs that had scorned us and the Anylookers who had judged us, fear and shame had become like a white noise machine that was always humming in the background of our lives. As our Stanford team delivered state-of-the-art PANS-mediated medical care to Anychild and swaddled our entire Anyfamily in a warm blanket of support and validation—for the first time in three years, the background noise began to abate.

As Anychild began to heal and life became quiet, the only sound left was Truth whispering gently, "I've got you . . . I've been right here all along."

PART TWO

NUTS AND BOLTS

In 2016, there were an estimated 162,000 children with PANS in the U.S. needing treatment, with scant resources to treat them. The vast majority of these families struggle to find care for their children, and face the same horrifying ignorance that we did during Anychild's hospitalization. There are not many physicians who are PANS-literate and complicating the matter further, many of the pediatricians that have heard of PANS question its legitimacy, due to the ongoing controversy that exists around the topic.

Where does this controversy come from? Well, there are without doubt a myriad of causes, but at the very heart of the issue is the utter paradigm shift that occurs when the notion is presented that some forms of mental illness are infection-based. This is a virtual game changer for medicine and the pharmaceutical industry as a whole.

I am not a medical doctor and my intention in writing about our experience is not to dole out one size fits all advice. My intent is to share what we have learned. And perhaps I can point out a few stones and help parents turn them over a bit earlier. Every child is unique, and every family's experience with this unenviable illness will be different. There are however, a few things that will be the same, and they are likely going to be these:

1) There is great risk that the Western Medical System will give your child only a few moments of its time before it delivers a one dimensional behavioral and/or psychiatric diagnosis. If you deflect that diagnosis, you will at first be met with the sympathetic response of a medical world that thinks you just need some time to come to terms with your child's diagnosis.

However, you will find that sympathy short lived if you continue to push beyond the behavioral/ psychiatric diagnosis for an answer. If you do not quickly accept the invitation you are given to join the tens of millions of other families that reside in the dank and frightening world of a pediatric psycho/behavioral diagnoses, the medical system will quickly fail you, shame you, and make it exceedingly hard for you to get care and treatment for your child.

2) The things that you will invariably investigate will require you to be strong willed and tough skinned, because the medical system, your neighbors, friends, loved ones, perhaps even your spouse, and the world at

large will not tolerate 'going there' with you. You will be questioned, you may be judged, you will be mocked, you will be pitied. Like we were, you may be accused of child abuse, or of having a mental illness of your own such as Munchausen by Proxy. If you want to make it through the fire, your three part mantra will have to become this:

What other people think is right for my Anychild is none of my business.

What other people think of me is none of my business.

What other people think of our Anyfamily is none of our business.

3) Remember this: Your goal is not to be liked or even to be understood. Your goal is to get an accurate diagnosis for your child and to move forward with the right treatment so that you can heal your child and reclaim your life.

Altering, changing, halting, or reversing whatever has happened inside your child will bring you to your knees: emotionally, socially, financially, and for some, spiritually. You will feel as if you have stepped into the wilderness, and in many ways, you have. But there are ways up this mountain . . . many, many ways up this mountain. I only know a handful of the many that are available, but it is my intention to share with you what I have learned and to inspire in you the impetus and fortitude to create new ways of your own.

LEARNING THE LINGO

At the time of this writing, there are a garden variety of diagnoses that likely fit into the topic of this book. Of course the most notable, and perhaps the most polarizing, is the premise of this book:

PANDAS stands for Pediatric Autoimmune Neuro-psychiatric **D**isorders **A**ssociated with **Strep**tococcal Infections. The term is used to describe a subset of children and adolescents who have Obsessive Compulsive Disorder (OCD) and/or tic disorders, and in whom symptoms worsen following infections such as Strep throat and Scarlet Fever.

PANS is a newer term used to describe the larger class of acute-onset OCD cases. **PANS** stands for Pediatric Acute-onset **Neuro-psychiatric S**yndrome, and includes all cases of abrupt onset OCD, not just those associated with streptococcal infections. (Some experts estimate that only ten percent of PANS/PANDAS diagnosed children have textbook

PANDAS.) Up to ninety percent of children affected
with PANS have GABHS (Strep) triggers, along with
a variety of accompanying triggers.

Some of the more well known non-strep triggers
for PANS are:

Mycoplasma Pneumonia
Pneumococcus (Streptococcus Pneumoniae)
Coxsackie B
Epstein Barr Virus
Lyme Disease
HHV-6 (Herpes Virus)

Autoimmune Encephalitis (AE) is a serious
medical condition in which the immune system
attacks the brain. It was mentioned in medical
literature as far back as the 1970s, but was at that
time considered an extreme rarity. It has only
recently become more well-known. One form of AE
known as Anti-NMDA Receptor Encephalitis was the
subject of the bestselling book *Brain on Fire* by
Susannah Cahalan. Anti-NMDA Receptor
Encephalitis occurs when antibodies produced by the
body's own immune system attack NMDA receptors
in the brain. NMDA receptors are proteins that
control electrical impulses in the brain. The
symptoms of AE are often nearly identical to those
seen with both PANDAS and PANS. (For the sake of
simplicity, the acronym of AE will not be included in

the remainder of this book, but its inclusion in all matters pertaining to PANS is implied.)

DIAGNOSIS

PANS itself is a clinical diagnosis, which means despite a name that brings to mind a cute little black and white bear, there is no black and white test available that gives a clean and irrefutable diagnosis.

Again I will turn to the National Institutes of Health to clarify the diagnosis. The diagnostic criteria used by the NIH are as follows:

- Presence of obsessive-compulsive disorder and/or a tic disorder
- Pediatric onset of symptoms (age three years to puberty)
- Episodic course of symptom severity (see information below)
- Association with group A Beta-hemolytic streptococcal infection (a positive throat culture for strep or history of scarlet fever)
- Association with neurological abnormalities (physical hyperactivity, or unusual, jerky movements that are not in the child's control)
- Very abrupt onset or worsening of symptoms

If the symptoms have been present for more than a week, blood tests may be done to document a current and/or preceding streptococcal infection.

In conjunction with the OCD and/or tics, most children with PANDAS/PANS will experience some combination of these symptoms as well:

- ADHD symptoms (hyperactivity, inattention, fidgeting)
- Separation anxiety (child is "clingy" and has difficulty separating from his/her caregivers. For example, the child may not want to be in a different room in the house from his/her parents.)
- Mood changes (irritability, sadness, emotional lability)
- Sleep disturbance
- Nighttime bed wetting and/or daytime urinary frequency
- Fine/gross motor changes (e.g., changes in handwriting)
- Joint pain

Anychild had been severely symptomatic for over one year when he was finally tested for strep. We have no way of knowing if he had an active strep infection during his onset, but in the year prior to his positive test, he had been in the throes of all the harrowing symptoms that are the hallmarks of PANS. Once he was diagnosed, we quickly found our way onto a pathway that was relatively clear-cut, although very difficult. Since his initial diagnosis, we have learned through subsequent flares that his body reacts to more than strep. This knowledge has changed his diagnosis to PANS.

Some may wonder how Anychild could have been sick with strep throat for so long and we did not know it. It can be confusing that strep can be present without a fever or sore throat. In a perfect world, when a child gets strep throat, those symptoms are present and the mystery is often solved with a rapid strep swab and a week's worth of Amoxicillin. A child with PANDAS does not get to live in that perfect world. Instead they get to live in the perfect storm, a storm that rages quietly in their nervous systems with nary a fever or sore throat anywhere in sight.

Strep is a wily opponent to say the least, and strep in the body of a child who is somehow predisposed to PANDAS is like an intruder that has learned how to disarm the child's immune response. Because it is a very ancient organism, it has learned through evolution how to hide within the human body. Strep evades the immune system for as long as possible by putting molecules on its cell wall that look nearly identical to molecules found in the heart, joint, skin and brain tissues. This is called "molecular mimicry" and allows the strep bacteria to escape detection for a time. This is also how rheumatic and scarlet fevers occur.

Once the strep bacteria are recognized as foreign to the body, the immune system begins to produce antibodies. Because of the molecular mimicry, the antibodies attack the authentic strep invaders *and* the 'clones' that were created through molecular mimicry. It is believed in PANDAS that these cloned cells have attached to the basal ganglia of the brain, and this in turn becomes a prime target for the immune attack. It is the attack on these clones that creates the firestorm known as PANDAS.

TREATMENT

At this time, these are the most widely accepted treatment options for PANS and PANDAS:

- Antibiotics
- Steroids
- IVIG
- Plasmaphoresus

ANTIBIOTICS

Antibiotics are a big part of the treatment protocol for PANDAS proper. Strep, when left untreated, can have dire consequences systemically and this is well known and respected.

The way that antibiotics are administered and used with PANS treatment is very different from other uses. It is imperative that Anyfamilies find PANS-literate medical care to assist them. There is no reason for me to write in any greater detail on this, as every PANS child is unique and will require an individualized, medically supervised treatment plan.

STEROIDS

Steroids are powerful drugs that have powerful side effects. It is well documented that short courses of steroids such as Prednisone can reduce and sometimes alleviate PANDAS symptoms all together. For most, steroids are a temporary fix, but new research indicates that long term, low dose, chronic steroids are a promising treatment for many children. Just the fact that PANS symptoms respond to steroids helps support the hypothesis that the symptoms are due to an inflammatory process.

The next listed treatment options require more explanation.

INTRAVENOUS IMMUNOGLOBIN

IVIG is the common acronym for Intravenous Immunoglobin. IVIG is used for many autoimmune illnesses and is not a new treatment or a treatment exclusive to PANS, by any means. IVIG is an intravenous blood product that is made from the immunoglobulin element of donor's blood. It takes approximately 1600 donors to produce one IVIG treatment. It works presumably by upgrading the dysfunctional immune system of the PANDAS patient. It is expensive, not without risk, and a very serious treatment modality. My understanding is that the majority of insurance carriers will not approve (pay for) PANDAS-related IVIG at this time. Thus far, Anychild's journey has spared us having to turn over this stone. I am glad it is there as an option, but thankful that we have not experienced it more intimately.

PLASMAPHORESUS or PLASMA EXCHANGE

(PEX) is the process of removing the harmful auto-antibodies from the blood system itself. This is, again, a complex, intricate, and expensive treatment procedure, and one we have been spared needing to consider.

As I write this book, there are more terms and names being used to describe sudden onset neuropsychiatric disorders in children. This expansion of verbiage will hopefully serve to negate the negative knee jerk reaction that many clinicians have to the term PANDAS (which means the onset of the disorder was brought on by a Group A strep infection).

For children like Anychild, this narrow, strep heavy definition fits only for what occurred at his onset. We have learned over the years that there are many, many other non-strep triggers that are just as valid and result in the same devastating and abrupt onset. It would be a tragedy for a poorly informed clinician to test a child for strep, and if the test is negative, stop the search there.

Viruses, Mycoplasma Pneumonia, and Lyme Disease are all well known and frequent triggers of the syndrome. There are many other known triggers, as well. If your child is unwell and you are investigating PANS as a possible cause, chances are you are going to have to fight to turn over this stone. Do your homework. This section of the book is to help you get started.

These disorders are complex neuro-psychiatric illnesses that continue to be subject to great debate within the traditional medical community. To worry about or waffle over what name to apply to what is happening to our children is something that parents like myself have no time for. To me, PANS describes the disorder as a whole, while PANDAS describes just one particular trigger that can cause the disorder.

PANS is an umbrella term that is not strep-specific, and with this broader scope, it can offer shelter to more families facing an inflammation-based, neuro-psychiatric illness. Anychild has PANS proper. We know that bacterial infections and viruses are what trigger the torrent of assaults on his nervous system.

But what about the millions of other children out there that have been labeled with a different acronym? The ones who have only been treated for behavioral and psychiatric symptoms? The ones with no fever and no sore throat who never get tested for infectious or bacterial culprits for sudden onset neuropsych symptoms? Most of the diagnoses that these children are given carry their very own acronym:

ADHD (Attention Deficit Hyperactivity Disorder)
ADD (Attention Deficit Disorder)
BPD (Bipolar Disorder)
IED (Intermittent Explosive Disorder)
ODD (Oppositional Defiant Disorder)
OCD (Obsessive Compulsive Disorder)
ASD (Autism Spectrum Disorder)
SPD (Sensory Processing Disorder) and many others.

In my journey to learn about PANS and heal Anychild, I heard doctors mention every single one of these as possible diagnoses for Anychild. During the acute portion of his illness, his symptoms bore such overlap with these other disorders that it became hard not to intuit that there is a link somewhere.

Could the bridges between *all of them* be inflammation and infection? And although a PANS diagnosis may get its initial shove from infection, could non-infection based inflammation caused by something else, such as a food allergy or an environmental factor, create neuro-psychiatric symptoms that cause children to roll down this same hill?

As I have said before, I am not a medical doctor, but in response to this question, common sense screams, "Why not?" And if you are an Anyparent trying to find your way through hell with your Anychild, I urge you to ask yourself the same question: "Why not?"

If you are the parent of a child who has been labeled with an acronym other than PANS, don't negate any of the information in this book, because your children's acronyms do not match Anychild's. I consider our journey and what we have learned about PANS to be applicable to a myriad of neuro-psychiatric disorders that today afflict so many of our children. These are the Shadow Syndromes that have yet to find their proper place in modern pediatric care.

This broad scope approach is simply adaptive on my part and not based on science proper, but I am willing to guess that if your child is on a fast track to hell like Anychild was, you don't really care what science proper has to say, because the medical community at large has turned a deaf ear to you and you are desperate for answers.

For the record, I am not so much interested in being 'right' as I am interested in sharing information with a broad audience that might find worth in our story. There are multitudes of parents today who are lost, with no hard diagnosis for what is happening to their children. They have been forced to traverse a difficult journey with a generation of children who face challenges unlike any generation before them.

My thoughts on this matter are simple: If the hallmarks of your experience include sudden onset neuro-psychiatric symptoms (sudden behavior changes, sudden sleep disruptions, sudden academic decline, sudden sensory issues, etc.), which then follow a saw tooth pattern of improvement and regression, your child may be suffering from an inflammation-based illness. If these symptoms are not static and enduring, seem to wax and wane due to factors you don't understand, the steps and information that apply to PANS that helped us may help you—even if PANS is not what your child has. There seems to be an umbrella covering a whole lot of children, and the storm they seek shelter from happens in their nervous systems—and inflammation is raining down.

If your child's process did not occur with an acute onset, but still includes neuro-psychiatric symptoms (sensory, behavioral, psychological, etc.), please don't stop reading. The simple terms I use to explain common features of PANS are perhaps inclusive of other infection/inflammation related neuro-psychiatric conditions, as well.

Today it is estimated that over ten million children in the United States are being prescribed stimulants, antidepressants and other psychotropic (mind altering) drugs for educational and behavioral problems. Of course, there are nuances and unique aspects to all of these conditions, but there is no argument that gives challenge to the fact that today's youth are suffering from an unprecedented number of disorders that were almost unheard of in prior generations.

PANDAS, PANS, Autoimmune Encephalitis (AE), NMDA Encephalitis, Children's Postinfectious Autoimmune Encephalopothy (CPAE) and the handful of other disorders which are similar, all have acute biological, neurological and psychiatric manifestations that then follow a saw tooth pattern of improvement and regression after onset. The current pediatric medical culture does not have any of these diagnoses, which are occurring in record numbers, on its radar.

I am well aware of the scientific process and how medical truth in our Western world is held to very specific standards. I respect this process. I have, however, always kept one eye on the fringe.

To me the fringe is that rough patch of road that sits just to the right and left of the carefully paved pathway of the scientific method. As a helping professional myself, I have seen miraculous things happen in the fringe. In science, these would be called 'anecdotal events,' because the results occur outside of controlled conditions.

In my own career and in the healthcare choices I have made for myself and our children, the fringe is not new territory. I have chosen many times to explore the fringe when working toward healing—but our experience with PANS was different. *PANS left us no choice but to go off road.* The conventional medical world had nothing to offer Anychild. Yes, psychiatric medications were offered and behavioral therapies were suggested, but that was the only direction that medical doctors wanted to go. And although early on I did not know what Anychild had, I knew intuitively that psychiatric drugs and cognitive behavioral therapies were not our answer.

In hindsight, I have to give my mother's gut credit. I know now that trying to use standard behavioral therapy with a child whose nervous system is on fire would have been like trying to douse an inferno with a squirt gun. When it comes

to medicating a PANDAS child with psychotropic
medications, PANDAS kids in general appear to be
unusually sensitive to the side effects of SSRIs and
other medications, and can have particularly bad
reactions to them. I am grateful for my choice to stay
off-road.

The things that helped Anychild were often in the
fringe. Even the antibiotics that finally dumbed down
Anychild's raging strep infection were in the fringe.
Yes, they were traditional medications, but they were
being used in a nontraditional way, which made our
regular medical doctors balk at their use (which is
overuse in their eyes.)

The things that helped Anychild were a pretty
short list that can be summed up in four words and
kept in chronological order: Diet, Diagnosis,
Treatment and Education. Finding our way to those
four seemingly common things was extraordinarily
difficult.

The steps that led us out of the wilderness of
PANS could be considered 'anecdotal' by science, but
these things, which are all in the fringe, have not
helped just our child. If it was only Anychild who had
been helped, I wouldn't write about them. There are
other PANDAS parents whose lead I have followed,
many thousands of them, who have found healing for
their children in these same unconventional areas.

Like me, they have fought tooth and nail for these
treatments because they knew this is what would
help to heal their children.

Medical science may not yet agree with us, but we have kept our eyes on those who walk a step ahead on the PANS path and we have taken notes. So, the following information may be 'anecdotal,' but if you are finding nothing for your child on the well traveled road of conventional medicine, it may be time to step into the fringe.

THE GLUTEN FREE/CASEIN FREE DIET

The first stone that I turned over in my quest to heal Anychild was the Gluten Free/Casein Free diet. Like everything else that I will discuss, this is considered controversial and there have been numerous 'scientific studies' done that will tell you there is not a link between diet and sudden onset neuro-psychiatric symptoms. In addition to this, there are scant studies that show that a vaccination can cause a neuro-psychiatric event such as Anychild experienced. The observations I have made are not based on studies. Rather, they are based on real life.

What I do know is that in early 2012, Anychild received three standard childhood vaccines. By mid-February, we were researching early onset mental illness due to the sudden and severe psychosis he developed. For six weeks nothing penetrated the horrible mental state that Anychild fell into.

Then we began a GF/CF diet. Within 24-hours we saw a change in him. Most scientific evidence shows that it takes weeks to months to fully see the effects of a GF/CF diet. This same science would likely say that 24-hours on a GF/CF diet could not drastically change anything in Anychild's biology.

I can't explain the science. I can only share the experience. Twenty-four hours of a GF/CF diet and we had our first significant breakthrough; many clinicians have told me that a change could not happen that quickly. It did. Hence, we began to feel the bumpy terrain of the fringe.

If you are a parent in the trenches of hell, science or not, the GF/CF diet is a stone well worth turning over. A major dietary change is not easy, but it can be the most potent medicine you can imagine in a child whose nervous system is suddenly firing wildly. I personally know of hundreds of parents who feel this is a very significant part of their child's healing from a Shadow Syndrome. And when I use the term GF/CF diet, I mean it in the strictest sense of the word. Not gluten light, not reducing dairy. I mean absolutely no gluten or casein, whatsoever. Both gluten and casein hide everywhere, so the vigilance that this diet takes is extreme. Every label must be scoured. Any food that is not hand cooked by you must be analyzed and picked apart for an ingredient list. One must learn that things like 'lactic acid' can mean the presence of casein, and that 'malt' contains gluten.

Anychild has fared exceedingly well with his diagnosis compared to many of his peers. I absolutely believe one of the reasons he has responded so well to his PANDAS treatment protocol, and has shown such resilience following his flares, is because six weeks into this nightmare we instituted the GF/CF diet and began to heal his gut. The gut and the brain are bedfellows, much more than most of us realize.

How exactly do gluten and dairy affect the brain? Well, it is a complex and sordid tale, and one I cannot possibly do justice to. What I can tell you is that our neuro-psychiatric health depends in large part on the neurotransmitters we can utilize.

Neurotransmitters are the chemicals that communicate information throughout our brain and body. It is estimated that over 100 million neurotransmitters line the length of the gut—approximately the same number as in the brain. This is why the term 'gut-brain' is starting to come into use. We virtually have a whole other brain in the belly. When the gut suddenly stops working like Anychild's did, the brain is essentially starved of those millions of neurotransmitters.

As I mulled over thoughts of how vaccines could have led to Anychild's sudden onset gluten intolerance, I began to better understand just how much gluten could have contributed to delusional behaviors as well. A chiropractor I took Anychild to early on alluded to this connection, and with the pieces of the puzzle starting to line up, a picture formed in my mind.

Imagine the gut continually producing millions of neurotransmitters that are ideally absorbed through the intestinal wall and then picked up by the bloodstream and carried up to the brain. The intestinal tract is lined with celia, tiny hairlike fingers that work to move these neurotransmitters and other things along. If one has Celiac Disease or reactivity to gluten, as soon as gluten is ingested, it causes all these hairlike celia to lie flat against the gut wall. The millions of celia lying flat creates a solid barrier that does not allow neurotransmitters, nutrients, and many other things through the gut lining.

I believe the vaccinations created an internal environment in Anychild that caused his celia to lay down hard and fast whenever he ingested gluten, and when that happened, he was essentially suddenly starved for many of the neuro-transmitters that he needed in order to live, think, and act normally. As I began to conceptualize my simplistic mental picture of what had happened in Anychild's gut, I felt like a blind woman who was slowly learning to read Braille. Things were beginning to make sense.

We followed a gluten-free, casein-free, nut-free, bean-free, preservative-free, dye-free diet like a religion for two years. It became the church we worshipped at. Diet was one of the few things within our control during the early days of our PANS adventure; and as difficult as adhering to the diet sometimes was, it was also very empowering.

I would never have willingly tested the efficacy of the GF/CF diet, but about six months into the diet, Anychild unknowingly got 'glutened.' After months of great behavior at school, on this particular day, Anychild had turned into a terror. At three o'clock recess he urinated on a child, hit another child in the head with a tire swing, and had multiple other instances of horrid behavior. I was crestfallen when I got the call from his school and they told me what had occurred. As we drove home in the car after school, Anychild expressed remorse for what he had done and said he did not know why he had behaved that way. Months before this, Anychild had begun to personify his Celiac Disease by acknowledging that when he ate 'bad foods' it woke up his 'bad brain' and when he ate 'good foods' it kept his good brain awake.

I asked him why he thought his 'bad brain' had woken up that day. His answer took me aback. "Maybe it was the new kind of pizza you gave me in my lunch." He went on to explain having eaten a piece of pepperoni pizza. I often packed GF/CF pizza in his lunch and I had that day. But pepperoni was not yet a food that Anychild could eat, so I knew that his piece of GF/CF pizza had gotten mixed up with another child's pepperoni pizza.

I was absolutely amazed that a lunchtime gluten and dairy ingestion could result in such radical behavior changes within hours. His behavior remained erratic for the following four days and then he resumed the level of behavioral functioning that we had become accustomed to.

If you are considering the GF/CF diet, there are a myriad of resources that you can use to assist you. There are cookbooks, phone apps, websites and support groups. Most restaurants now have many GF dining options and are willing to work with patrons to assure that your meal remains GF/CF.

Some children, like Anychild, respond very quickly to the GF/CF diet. For others, improvement may be slower. I have read that it should be tried for a full two months in order to ascertain its efficacy, but remember that this requires two months of absolute, unfailing GF/CF eating.

The blood tests that were ordered on Anychild to gauge the level of his reaction to gluten offered us the first biological proof that there was an attack happening in his system. The presence of antibodies gave us an objective look at his reactions and made the gluten issue tangible. There are many antibody specific tests that a well versed practitioner can order. If you are unable to find a resource, you may want to do a search in your local area for doctors who practice either Functional Medicine or Integrative Medicine. I have found, far and away, that chiropractors are the most willing and the most knowledgeable about this.

It is important to note that when we become highly reactive to one substance, such as gluten, our system can then become oversensitive. Often times this will cause what Functional Medical doctors call a cross reaction. This means the body in a heightened state of awareness reacts to other foods that would normally be tolerated. Dairy tends to have a very common cross reaction, as does soy. Anychild had a variety of cross reactions: dairy, soy, and chocolate were the strongest. Because his system has been quieted down by the strict GF/CF diet, we were able to reintroduce chocolate into his diet about sixteen months after we began. At the two-year point, we were able to add in everything but gluten.

Although Anychild has been deemed 'Celiac,' I maintain hope that there is some wiggle room for improvement. The formal diagnostic process for Celiac is complex, with the gold standard for diagnosis being a small-bowel biopsy that shows characteristic histologic abnormalities. That is an invasive, costly, and potentially dangerous procedure that we don't care to embark upon with Anychild. The more common diagnostic criteria often used include:

- Subsequent improvement (clinical and/or histologic) on a gluten-free diet
- Laboratory findings that show Celiac disease-associated antibodies

- Presence of Celiac Disease-associated human leukocyte antigen (HLA) alleles, a Celiac-specific gene

Whether it was fortunate or unfortunate, Anychild met all three of these criteria. The only piece of the puzzle remaining was the small bowel biopsy. Not only did we not care to put Anychild through this, his life and its improvement sans gluten was proof that living GF was powerful medicine for him.

I have tried to understand the differences between the genetic components that lead to Celiac Disease proper, and those that cause the body to mount an immune response against gluten, but this has been difficult and mindbending for this Anymom.

Genetic testing confirmed that Anychild was born with half of the DQ2 heterodimer, which is one of the genetic markers for Celiac Disease. This produced an official (and very confusing) test result of 'Positive for Celiac Disease Associated HLA allele.'

Even my layman's brain could deduce that this was a murky diagnosis, and HLA alleles-talk made little sense to me. I researched and learned that an allele is one aspect of a gene, which results in a hereditary change. So Anychild had half of one of these. I learned to look at these test results as 'Anychild possessed half of the recipe for Celiac.'

This alone intrigued me a great deal. Since he had spent the first five years of his life happily munching on Wheat Thins®, coexisting with this 'half recipe for Celiac,' what the hell had happened? As I began to explore and understand more about the field of Epigenetics, my wonder morphed into dismal understanding.

Epigenetics is the study of how the environment or other outside forces can cause a previously unexpressed gene to begin expressing. We do not believe that Anychild was reactive to gluten prior to his vaccinations. I do not state this as a fact, because he could very well have been reacting to gluten in a much more subtle way, not yet causing symptoms we noticed.

After the vaccinations, he became acutely neurologically ill. The first intervention that made a noticeable difference in him was the removal of gluten from his diet.

In Epigenetics talk, something (maybe the vaccine, maybe something else) caused his previously unexpressed Celiac allele to start screaming. Prior to this, if it was awake, it was just whispering. Anychild had half the genetic marker for Celiac, this was fact; but something definitely caused it to kick into high gear, seemingly overnight.

Anychild's genetic testing was certainly supportive of, at the very least, an immune response to gluten, but there were other laboratory findings that seemed to shore up the results, which were significant to his PANS physicians. Those blood tests that the helpful chiropractor ordered early on, just after Anychild's onset, showed that Anychild was positive for several tissue transglutaminase antibodies. These are antibodies directed against an enzyme normally present in the intestines called 'tissue transglutaminase' or tTG.

With Celiac Disease, the body produces two types of antibodies that attack tTG: immunoglobulin A (IgA) and immunoglobulin G (IgG). The presence of form A indicates an immune response being directed toward the intestines, whereas the presence of form G correlates to an immune attack being directed toward the nervous system/brain. Anychild had both types of these antibodies circulating in his system during those early days when he was lost to us, when we had no idea what had happened to him.

We still don't really know if Anychild fits the 'formal criteria' for Celiac Disease, but at this point, it really is just semantics. Celiac as a label is not something we embrace, but being gluten free has been a potent form of healing in his system.

That being said, becoming gluten free at the age of five is a long haul. I am still hopeful that at some point Anychild may be able to one day tolerate at least small amounts of gluten. When I am feeling particularly hopeful, I have reasoned that perhaps that damn half Allele that 'turned on' so suddenly in 2012 will be coaxed into 'turning off' one day. I have also entertained the thought that perhaps what Anychild has is more like an allergy, one that he can grow out of in the future. I had many food allergies as a child that I have transcended in adulthood. I keep my fingers crossed, wishing this same thing for Anychild.

This hope propelled me into researching food allergies and how they might contribute to neurological issues. When I brought this concept up to traditional doctors, I was quickly dismissed and told that food allergies did not and could not correlate to neurological changes. But when I researched the topic on my own, what I learned was nothing short of amazing.

I was introduced to the work of Dr. Doris Rapp, a board certified Environmental Medical Specialist and Pediatric Allergist. She is also a homeopath. She served as Clinical Assistant Professor Emeritus of Pediatrics at the State University of New York at Buffalo until January 1996. I was absolutely floored by the decades old film clip I watched (from the Phil Donohue Show to be exact) showing children before and after eating foods they were allergic to.

The footage is stunning. The overt changes that occur in these children within minutes of eating the offending food are extreme and I would encourage any of you who may doubt the power that food can have on our neurological/emotional and/or behavioral health to do a search for these videos. They truly speak for themselves.

I am not a gastroenterologist, allergist or
nutritionist. I am just an Anymom who knows that
gluten is a weapon of mass destruction in my child's
system. Taking it out of his diet has changed his life.
It has changed ours. Living gluten free is not simple
or cheap, but it is achievable and its effect has been
nothing short of magical. If you are in the trenches, I
urge you to learn more about this topic and proceed
in the direction that feels right for your child.

LABORATORY TESTING

If you think your child may have PANS, blood
work is essential. Most traditional practitioners will
not routinely run the tests that are specific to rooting
out PANDAS/ PANS. You have to ask for them. The
specific blood work that was run on Anychild that led
to his PANDAS diagnosis (that later became PANS)
included these labs:

- Anti-Streptolysin O Titers
- Anti-DNase Titers
- Streptozyme
- Mycoplasma Pneumoniae IgG and IgM
- Lyme Western Blot and/or Igenex
- IgG, IgA and IgM Levels
- IgE Level
- IgG Subclasses IgG1, IgG2, IgG3 and IgG4
- Vitamin D (25-OH)
- Pneumococcal Antibody Panel (14 serotypes)

- CBC with Differential and Platelets
- Babesia, Bartonela, Ehrlichia Titers
- Coxsackie A Titers
- EBV Panel
- Coxsackie B Titers
- Parvovirus B-19 Titers
- HHV-6 Titers
- CMV Titers
- CMP
- MTHFR

There are others, but these are the basic tests that will likely be helpful as you investigate.

Some children are considered to have PANDAS or PANS without positive blood work. This is an area of considerable debate and it is a complex subject. How do strep, other bacteria and viruses achieve that thing called 'molecular mimicry,' which allows them to go undetected by blood tests and perhaps to cross the blood/brain barrier? In laymen's speak, this means that the bad guys (strep, etc.) can go undercover and remain undetected by the immune system, even though they have set up house and are thriving.

Anychild's initial blood work showed high levels of active strep, as well as high IgG and IgM immune assays for Mycoplasma Pneumonia, Epstein Barr Virus and HHV-6 (Herpes), indicating both acute and past infections. With long-term antibiotic and antiviral medications, the antibody levels have come down. The year following his onset was likely one long PANS flare, and since his diagnosis in March of 2013, he has had three very serious flares, where his original symptom set returned.

The first flare included strep and EBV and HHV-6. The second appeared to be triggered solely by the viruses EBV and HHV-6, unless the process of molecular mimicry allowed the strep bacteria to remain hidden, when it was actually active. The third was caused by strep and Influenza B that unfortunately arrived together and resulted in both his brain and his muscles being attacked by his immune system.

Chasing these infections with blood work quickly becomes a cloak and dagger operation. In our world, bacteria and viruses have taken on almost human characteristics as we track them and they learn to evade our efforts. *All of this stems from a compromised immune system that is at the heart of PANS and PANDAS.*

In 2013, a PANS-specific blood test by Moleculara Labs came out. It is called the Cunningham Panel. The Cunningham Panel consists of a series of five assays and although not considered 'diagnostic' in nature, it does offer important insight into how anti-neuronal antibodies play a key role in PANDAS and other illnesses like it.

Anychild's Cunningham Panel showed a variety of positive indicators for PANS, but perhaps most telling were the very high CaM Kinase II levels. This is a multifunctional enzyme highly concentrated in the brain that works in neurotransmission and neuronal excitability. I have heard many doctors verbalize their thoughts that high CaM Kinase II levels seem to be one of the smoking guns in the PANS puzzle.

Anychild's Cunningham Panel was patently positive for the markers believed to be most indicative of PANS, offering strong support for the diagnosis he had already been given. This reaffirmed for us that we had found the correct path to follow for his healing. These high levels of anti-neuronal antibodies that the Cunningham Panel showed in Anychild's bloodstream continued to expunge the dirty 'Medical Child Abuse' smear that an Anylooker had left on our world months before.

The Cunningham Panel is not always covered by insurance and should be considered on an individual basis. Do your own research and talk to your doctor to see if it seems to be applicable to your situation.

UNDERSTANDING OBSESSIVE COMPULSIVE (OCD) and TIC DISORDERS

The heart-wrenching cornerstones of PANS are the obsessions, compulsions and tics that show up seemingly overnight.

Anychild's OCD behaviors were atypical compared to many. Often with PANS, there are obsessions related to cleanliness, germs, bowel and bladder elimination, intrusive thoughts, and severe dietary restrictions. These symptoms are overwhelming and completely disable all sense of normalcy.

At onset, Anychild did not display any OCD in relation to cleanliness, germs, or his bowel and bladder habits, although with his third flare (two years after diagnosis), he erupted into all of these with a vengeance. At his initial onset, we did see a drastic eruption of OCD behaviors that were centered around his eating rituals, and his need to collect things and store them in a certain way and in a specific order.

His thinking became rigid and unyielding. Food had to be placed a certain way on the plate, he had to be served what he wanted before he asked for it, and in the way he wanted it to be. If we incorrectly intuited what his dietary compulsion was in the moment, it would result in a rage that sent food flying at us and across the room. It was exasperating and completely irrational.

Meal times became unbearable for all of us. And it was not just his food placement that became an issue. His food intake became grossly constricted as well. From onset, until we began the GF/CF diet six weeks later, Anychild would only eat two foods, and if he was not given those foods, he flatly refused to eat anything at all.

As fate would have it, those two foods were whole wheat brownie bars, and liquid yogurt. Remember, at onset we did not know that what was happening to Anychild was propelled by wheat and dairy. To add further fuel to the fire that was burning within Anychild, the drinkable yogurt he was consuming by the dozens each day, contained a strain of the strep bacteria among its yogurt cultures. (I had learned that when a probiotic has the initial 's' in front of it, it stands for Streptococcus.) We were essentially feeding the beast a perfect diet. In doing so, we were allowing the beast to grow bigger, while the child we loved faded farther and farther from our grasp.

At onset, when I was cornered into conversation by others regarding Anychild's limited dietary intake, I commonly got the glib reply that I should hold my parental ground in front of a plate of broccoli and once Anychild got hungry enough, he would eat it. That is an easy philosophy to dispense when not walking in our shoes. Anychild would go three-quarters of the day with no food or water intake as it was.

We had already bypassed any sense of having control over what was happening. Luckily, we let go of the hope that Anychild would imbibe in a nutrient dense food plan. It simply was not a battle we waged with him.

In retrospect, I am glad. Unbeknownst to us at the time, many children afflicted with PANS can suffer symptoms of anorexia as well. He restricted his food choices immensely, but at least Anychild continued to eat.

Even though I have a strong background in the mental health field, at onset I did not realize that Anychild's behaviors were reflective of OCD. After all, he was my child, not my client, so I did not view him through eyes seeking clinical indicators of a disorder. I suspect many parents whose child is afflicted with PANS must feel the same exasperation that we did at first.

As parents we experienced Anychild as demanding, unyielding, selfish, self-centered, and unreasonable. We did not see that he was suffering from Acute Onset OCD. We learned that when his foods were not arranged the way he wanted them on the plate, he felt like he was going to die. We did not know that the reason he became so violent and rage filled if one of his dollar bills had a crease in it, was because he felt like a bomb would erupt inside of him if they were not all perfectly flat and aligned.

The rages that at first seemed to indicate that we had a bad child and/or that we were bad parents, were simply unpreventable. There was no plan that we could engage in that would allow the world to arrange itself in a way that did not set Anychild off.

Before we realized this grim truth, we tried to reason with him, we tried time out, we began to slam

our fists on the counter and yell. We realized that the
only compassionate thing we could really do was to
separate ourselves from his unbending demands and
let the rage happen.

The rages were simply unstoppable. It was not a
matter of if, but when. Over time we began to see
these daily rages as necessary events that somehow
let steam out of his system. This theory began to
make even more sense when we learned about
Sensory Processing Disorder or SPD.

As far as Anychild having tics, the predominant
symptom he displayed was sudden onset stuttering,
which later resolved. A number of people have
suggested that children with Tourette's Syndrome
may have a higher frequency of stuttering than seen
in the general population. This has raised the
possibility of a causal link between the two disorders,
especially because there are suggestions that children
and adults who stutter may have atypical functioning
of the basal ganglia, which is the primary area of the
brain presumed to be affected by PANS.

The literature reports the incidence of stuttering
in Tourette's Syndrome ranging from seven percent
to as high as thirty-three percent. Tourette's is one of
the primary misdiagnoses made among children
afflicted with PANS. After Anychild was diagnosed
with PANDAS and we became mindful of tics, we
were surprised at how many he did display and only
during flares. They were subtle, but very definite

repetitive patterns of movement that we had not
previously noticed.

SENSORY PROCESSING DISORDER

One of the hallmarks of PANS is sudden onset
sensory disorders. At onset, Anychild became acutely
sensitive to almost everything in his world. He could
not tolerate light, sound or texture. He wore only
three shirts, all mock turtle necks made from a very
smooth nylon type of material. He could only tolerate
loose fitting silky sweatpants and his predominant
color choice was black: black shoes, black socks, etc.
His Occupational Therapist later told us that his
clothing choices indicated he was displaying *tactile-
defensiveness.* His extreme sensitivity to sound and
light were indicative of a nervous system that could
not properly route the many forms of stimuli that our
senses continually take in.

His sudden onset extreme hyperactivity was
likely indicative of what is called *sensory seeking
behavior.* He basically needed to be frenetically active
at all times. He could not sit still, play a board game,
quietly watch TV, or look at a book. He was in
constant motion. Thankfully, Anychild's predominant
strength seems to be an athletic-like agility. He has
excellent hand/eye coordination, and throughout his
onset and subsequent months of PANS-related
behaviors, he remained active in a multitude of

sports. He was often not able to attend to rules, or follow through with team drills, etc., but his actual physical skills remained sharp, which was essential to his sense of self-esteem.

If your child exhibits sensory issues, often the best way to work through these issues is with an Occupational Therapist. We learned essential ways to calm Anychild's senses using movement, pressure, texture, sound, and light in ways that soothed, rather than irritated his system. An amazing number of things become 'medicinal' when you step into the fringe.

MTHFR AND GENETICS

During our very first visit to the specialist who diagnosed Anychild's PANS, this doctor predicted that Anychild would have a set of genetic mutations called MTHFR. I remember presuming he was wrong. Anychild had been robustly healthy his entire life.

How could a child who had a fever only once in his life have genetic mutations? Well, as you already know, I was wrong. The official name of this gene is "Methylenetetrahydrofolate reductase (NAD (P)H)."

When there is a defect in the MTHFR gene, it disrupts the body's ability to process folic acid and/or folate. This, in turn, is believed to promote high levels of homocysteine levels in the blood, which can then negatively affect mental health and mood.

This inability to process folic acid (vitamin B9) can have serious effects on not just cognition and mood regulation, but also the body's ability to process and excrete toxins.

My ability to gene speak is very limited, so I will keep it simple. Anychild has some common MTHFR mutations, paired with some less common mutations that could make it difficult for him to properly utilize B vitamins. This likely affects his emotional, behavioral, and physical symptoms.

These mutations *also* cause a breakdown in his ability to detoxify his body of certain things. Physicians have told me, and research indicates that children that have both MTHFR mutations (as well as others) are particularly vulnerable to vaccine reactions. If this fringe information is true, imagine the lives that could be changed with this knowledge. If Anychild had received one vaccination at a time, instead of three, life may have proceeded forward very differently for Anychild. Something as simple as a delayed vaccine schedule could make a critical difference in the lives of millions.

There are specific protocols for addressing MTHFR mutations. These relatively simple, supplement and nutrition-based protocols help bypass the detox pathways that are not working and allow the body to function more optimally. Many PANS children have detoxification issues; many parents have found that identifying and treating them is essential to the healing process.

After learning about Anychild's MTHFR issue, we had further genetic testing done, which gave us other important pieces of his biological puzzle. We utilized a simple and economical genetic test called 'The 23andMe.' This test offers a host of interesting information, about ancestry and many health issues, but what we really wanted to know was specific to his methylation and detoxification issues.

The 23andMe results showed us a variety of Anychild's Single Nucleotide Polymorphisms (SNP) (pronounced 'snip'). SNPs are genetic changes in which a single base in the DNA differs from the usual base at that position. As fate would have it, Anychild had a number of very significant SNPs. It is too complex for me to articulate properly here, but due to the large number of SNPs Anychild had, I began to investigate further.

My seeking took me to the work of Dr. Amy Yasko. Dr. Yasko's work is reputable and successful, but is still considered to be in the fringe. Among other things, her work has contributed meaningful information to the management of SNPs in relation to chronic inflammation, and immunological and neurological disorders. She has achieved considerable success in halting and in some cases reversing the effects of debilitating diseases, including ALS, MS, Parkinson's Disease, Alzheimer's Disease, SLE,

Myasthenia Gravis and Autism. Her most recent focus is her program to help reverse Autism.

As I delved into her work, I saw that many of the SNP's that she has identified as problematic and possibly contributory to Autism Spectrum Disorders (ASDs) were the very SNPs that Anychild had.

What I have not divulged prior to now, but is important to state, is that Anychild had only one other vaccination at the age of six months, prior to the set he received at five years of age. He had such a violent reaction at six months, I delayed all further shots until I was required to get them when he began kindergarten.

I believe the thousands of parents who say that their children were normal and began showing signs of Autism only after their vaccinations. I know that many scientific sources debunk this.

But I live in the fringe, where life does not always match up to what government, pharmacy, or the gods of science claim as facts.

I often wonder what would have happened to Anychild if he had received the recommended 49 doses of fourteen different vaccines, prior to the age of six. The thought of this sickens me when I reflect on what three vaccines produced when he was a healthy, happy, 40-pound, five-year-old. The shots he got that day were supposed to be given to him between the ages of fourteen and eighteen months. I reiterate: It was not the shots that caused the problems. It was Anychild's biochemistry in relation to the shots that made our perfect storm.

I cannot state strongly enough that I am not anti-vaccine. I do believe that for certain children, a delayed vaccination schedule, along with 'greener' vaccines (making the carriers and preservatives used in them less toxic) would be a wonderful start to a happier ending for everyone. I also believe that the individual biochemistry of children should be taken into account with vaccine schedules, and with tests available like the 23andMe and others, this is a viable direction in which to proceed to possibly safeguard the health of children in relation to vaccines.

A predominant number of children who have PANS have MTHFR issues, and a handful of other SNPs that are common. It is also very standard knowledge among PANS parents that our children fare horribly with vaccines. Our story of onset beginning shortly after a vaccine is not uncommon, and many other PANS children have suffered horrible flares and setbacks after receiving vaccines or flu mist. It is a precarious issue, rife with extreme controversy, but we are talking about children's lives and well-being. We owe it to our children to keep turning stones over until we have more answers.

Learning about Anychild's genetic makeup and where his detoxification pathways have failed him has been heady, difficult work. I am a neophyte in my

understanding, but the knowledge I have gained has
been invaluable. By using the information gained
with The23andMe and relying on the assistance of
geneticists and PANS medical professionals to wade
through the results with me, I have been empowered
as a parent. From understanding his SNPs, I have
learned some concrete things about foods, medicines,
and environmental agents that can all behave
differently in Anychild's system due to his unique
genetic makeup. Today we live life around them. This
genetic knowledge is kind of like having a compass in
hand while we poke around, out here in the fringe.

INFLAMMATION AND DETOXIFICATION

If there are two things that have truly become a
way of life in our house they are these: reducing
inflammation and promoting detoxification. Both of
these things are at the foundation of Anychild's
struggles. One of the very first treatment approaches
our PANS physician recommended was daily use of
an anti-inflammatory. The most familiar of these was
ibuprofen. Soon after diagnosis, we began giving
Anychild three daily sizeable doses of Advil. He
improved. This provided immediate real time proof
that what we were dealing with was inflammation-
based.

Now, we use Advil only when we see symptoms
and behaviors that we now know are inflammation

triggered. Although Ibuprofen can be hard on the gastrointestinal tract, when we have maintained the schedule recommended by our PANS team, we have had no issues. This is a simple, relatively safe, and available over the counter treatment option—but be warned, if you speak it out loud, you are going to end up in the fringe.

There are many other anti-inflammatories that we have used with good success. Turmeric, or its active ingredient Curcumin, is a potent anti-inflammatory supplement that is reportedly effective for many. Omega-3 Fatty Acids, Medium Chain Triglyceride Oil, and Flax Oil also have anti-inflammatory properties that seem helpful to many.

As soon as we realized the gluten/Celiac link with Anychild, we began instituting an 'anti-inflammatory' lifestyle. We eliminated all trans fats, all processed meat, nuts, beans, dairy, refined oils such as safflower, corn and sunflower oils, all artificial food additives like aspartame and monosodium, dyes, preservatives, and anything else with a name I could not spell or pronounce.

We no longer used sunscreens that had any toxic chemical ingredients in them, nor did we use mosquito repellant, air fresheners, or any home cleaning products that were toxic in any way. Anychild began sleeping on organic white cotton sheets, and we tried to minimize his consumption of foods that were in plastic or aluminum containers. I bought new nontoxic cookware, and I learned to sneak anti-inflammatory foods in wherever and whenever I could.

Today we no longer have to live within the confines of such a restrictive way of life. Gluten is the only food that we religiously avoid, although we still eat clean and keep Anychild as unburdened as possible by removing anything toxic that could come either through diet or environment.

GHOSTS

During our years as an Anyfamily, there were times when people looked at me like I was crazy because I so closely monitored what came into Anychild's world. As a PANS mom, I know of no other way to live. Anyfamilies fear the unknown future and they are constantly drawn backwards toward the ghosts of the past. It has become obvious to clinicians that many PANS families suffer symptoms of Post Traumatic Stress Disorder (PTSD.)

Whole family PTSD is a very real occurrence with PANS. It is a group activity of the worst kind, where a current stressor sends one's fight or flight system into overdrive, based on an old memory that resembles something currently happening. Family members then careen into one another with their emotional reactions the way bumper cars bounce around at amusement parks.

Because you know that an exacerbation can loom on the horizon at any given moment, it is hard to not always be on guard. One case of strep throat in the classroom and it is almost impossible for an Anyparent not to be braced for a return to hell. We know how quickly the light in our Anychildren can grow dark; it is hard not to live a somewhat germ phobic life.

Prior to PANS, there was nary a germaphobe to be found in our Anyfamily. We had lived the five-second rule and flourished (the one that if you drop food on the ground but pick it up quickly, it is not really dirty). After PANS routed through our world and turned everything upside down, germ warfare became a very serious part of life.

If someone in our social circle was ill, plans were changed, and commitments cancelled. We even learned to be wary of those around us who had received recent 'live vaccines,' because the recipients 'shed' the virus strain that was used to create the live, attenuated vaccine for a period of time. Intranasal flu mist was the live vaccine we became wary of when we learned that the shedding was capable of setting off Anychild's immune system. Anychild would not get the flu, but his immune system would react to the virus around him and set off mild flare symptoms.

Anychild had a heightened sense of awareness around germs, as well. If a friend borrowed his clothing, Anydad and I would have to talk him off the 'contamination cliff' that his mind would almost instantly create. Because he knew what happened inside of his body when his immune system was tipped off, he became more and more germ defensive in the way he lived his life.

Luckily for us, this presented in a functional way. He became a consummate hand washer, but never to the point of excess.

Hyper-vigilance is exhausting, but unavoidable for Anyfamilies. To this day, whenever Anychild's behavior spikes just a little bit, we brace for that free fall into the abyss that we know could come. When Anychild feels sick, or his throat feels scratchy, his fear is palpable. He knows that the same illness that might earn his classmates no more than a few days out of school and a batch of chicken soup, could send him tumbling straight down the dark rabbit hole of PANS.

It's a very unenviable way to live. I have friends, and some ex-friends, who likely find me hyper-vigilant and excessive in my attentiveness to the nuances of Anychild's life. If he wakes during the night with a nightmare, I do not sleep again that night. I am much too busy planning my counterattack for what I know might be coming. If he sniffles or says his throat feels scratchy, I pull out all the stops on keeping him warm, hydrated, and full of virus and bacteria reducing supplements and foods. I white knuckle it through the next few days, watching him like a hawk, waiting for any sign that the enemy has reappeared on the horizon of our life.

The descent into a PANS flare is often rapid and harrowing, so much so that one very experienced PANS clinician has coined the term the 'Exorcist Syndrome' to describe what he has observed. The 'Exorcist Syndrome' symptom list includes:

- Hyper Acute Onset: Parents can often pinpoint the hour of change.
- Ballistic Tics: Forceful, unrestrained, violent movements; i.e., they can appear seizure like, can be violent to self and others. They may hit, bite, intend to maim.
- Disinhibition: Expletives, little to no impulse control, severe behavioral acting out.
- Falsetto Vocal Changes: Voice is clear, no aphasia, but there is a drastic change to the quality of the voice, which becomes gruff, demonic, high pitched, infantile, etc.
- Symptoms seem to turn on and off like a switch.

So the fact that a PANS physician has coined the term the 'Exorcist Syndrome' to describe a PANS onset should speak volumes about why PANS families suffer from PTSD and behave in ways that the world does not always understand.

For those who have mocked us for our vigilance with Anychild: I will defend this by saying that when you have taken the very rapid descent into PANS hell, it is very, very hard not to spend the rest of your days guarding against it.

To those who find mothers like me overprotective, obsessive, or just irritating: I have nothing to say, other than I hope you NEVER have to strap on your boots and come onto the battlefield where I walk every day.

To the Anydoctors who listened to our tale and offered no more than a sympathetic smirk as I described what I believed was happening inside Anychild: When the validation of this illness becomes mainstream, I hope this will soften you. I hope you will care for the Anyfamilies you meet in the future with compassion, so they never feel the humiliation and shame that we felt in your offices.

To the Anylookers of this world: Before you go forth into the world and accuse, be bold enough to ask direct questions. And after you have asked the questions, *be brave enough to listen to the answers.* PANS is a heavy burden to bear, but ignorance is even heavier.

Anylookers are an unfortunate consequence of the dynamic PANS creates. The simple truth is that when you are navigating through your life with this unpredictable illness living under your roof, it fundamentally changes the way you move through the world. The people around you pick up on this.

When Anylookers are curious but not open, they take it upon themselves to fill in the blanks on their own. They piece together bits of information and they compare it to what they believe is right and normal and, "V*oila!*" Things do not line up.

The isolation we have felt and the criticism we have endured is not unique. We have learned firsthand through Anychild's medical team at Stanford that the 'Medical Child Abuse' allegation we endured is one many other Anyfamilies have faced, as well. This fact is a dismal reminder of just how skewed the unbaptised public's perception of PANS can be.

The simple black and white truth of a PANS diagnosis is that it permeates every aspect of a family's life, and it puts you at odds with those around you. When your child has PANS, things are never going to line up the way they do in other people's lives.

And those who observe and judge how an Anyfamily does or does not move through the medical system truly know nothing at all about what this experience is like. Figuring out how to make your way toward medical care with a PANS child is like walking through a minefield. Every step you take has the potential to destroy whatever progress you may have made, and every turn not taken could have been the one that opened a door that changed everything.

When you have a flaring PANS child, stepping into a medical facility or a doctor's office that is not PANS aware is not just terrifying—it can be life altering. All PANS parents know we run the risk of encountering an uninformed physician who can make a unilateral decision to treat our Anychildren as if they are mentally ill. Parental rights are a thin branch, but many parents who are blessed with normal, healthy children do not know this. Any parent of a PANS child knows what it feels like to be forced to tiptoe out onto that skinny branch with their Anychildren flailing wildly in their arms. You learn to be discreet and you learn to walk a very big circle around a medical system that does not understand your world.

Anyparents live in a world that other parents would not wish on even their worst enemies. The toll that it takes on parents as individuals is monumental. Maintaining our Anychildren's health becomes an all consuming priority. Marital strife runs high and often there is disagreement between parents on treatment choices and medical care. If the dynamic is complicated by divorce, the stakes become even higher.

Thankfully, Anydad and I had always been on the same page. Although our stressors were incredibly high, we gave the Anylookers in our world every opportunity to learn the intricacies of our PANS journey, and we maintained the integrity of our marriage. In the end, what we were left with was a stronger marriage and a tight knit and supportive inner circle of loved ones who took the time to understand PANS and give Anychild the love and assistance he needed.

The importance of having a support system that understands the PANS journey cannot be overstated. One of my hopes in writing this book is that it will be shared and used to educate, to help PANS families build bridges with those around them. Family members and social circles who understand the nature of PANS are necessary supports that every family needs. Those who ask questions and inform themselves become advocates and sources of support.

We have learned to beware of the curious kind of folk who exist on the fringe of our world: the Anylookers who gawk from a distance, but will not ask questions. These dangerous Anylookers become one more source of pain for families already living with unimaginable, invisible burdens.

When education and information about PANS and all of the other shadow syndromes facing our children really begins to flow, and the reality of these hellish disorders sets in, compassion will replace ignorance. *There simply can be no other outcome for our Anychildren.*

OUT OF THE SHADOWS

PANS cannot hide when you know how to look for it. And it is a disorder that follows an astonishingly predictable path. With early treatment, outcomes are excellent and long-term effects are significantly minimized. Our story is about PANS, but of course it is not just about PANS. It is equally about the vast array of these Shadow Syndromes—these neuro-psychiatric ills that are rampant among Anychildren today.

We have a generation of children that are clothed in acronyms: ADHD (Attention Deficit Hyperactivity Disorder), ASD (Autism Spectrum Disorder), OCD (Obsessive Compulsive Disorder), SPD (Sensory Processing Disorder), PANDAS (Pediatric Autoimmune Neuro-Psychiatric Disorder Associated with Strep A), PANS (Pediatric Autoimmune Neuro-psychiatric Syndrome), ODD (Oppositional Defiant Disorder), IED (Intermittent Explosive Disorder), BPD (Bipolar Disorder)—and the list goes on and on.

I never planned on being an activist and when Anychild is gifted with consecutive months of blissful, symptom free health, I am still sometimes tempted to turn away from the PANS world and not look back. But that's what I had done prior to Anychild's admission to the hospital. When I took my eyes off the beast, it emerged and cornered us in a hospital system with not a single PANS-literate physician to lean toward. PANS tossed Anychild into the air the same way Anychild had tossed that silly plastic paratrooper after his dental appointment—and we landed with the same sickening thud.

This last thud, the hospitalization and subsequent needless battle for antibiotics that sent our world and our social system into chaos, was the final impetus for me to put pen to paper and write this book. For the length of a 25-year career as a helping professional, the main thrust of my work has been as a writer and an educator.

I have a practice specialty that I love and it is worlds away from anything even hinting at pediatric neuro-psychiatric disorders. I do not want to be a spokesperson for this illness, but I do want this book to be a voice. PANS has been a life altering experience for our family. Sharing our story and providing insight and education to others is a way for us to make meaning out of what we have been through.

Some readers may question the authenticity of this book, due to the anonymous nature of this writing, and wonder why I have written under the pen name of Anymom.

There are several reasons, but the main one is our desire to keep Anychild's identity obscure. PANS is only part of his story. It is not who he is, nor is it a place we want him to linger one moment more than he has to. By the time this book goes to press, he will have spent more than five years of his life navigating through a controversial illness. Years have been lost to this beast, social relationships have been shattered, and tens of thousands of dollars have been spent. Our preference is to not give one more thing up to PANS.

Another draw toward anonymity is simple weariness. As a family, living in the midst of a controversial illness is exhausting. For every ounce of support we have gleaned, we have been pummeled with a pound of criticism. Sharing our story with a larger audience was never an easy decision, *but this book exists as much to support the Anyfamilies as it does to quiet all of the Anylookers.*

One of my favorite writers, Brene Brown, says, "If you are not in the arena also getting your ass kicked, I am not interested in your feedback." The Anylookers of this world jeer from the cheap seats. If the Anyfamilies like us do not speak up and tell our stories, the Anylookers of this world will continue to see only what their small, dimly lit peepholes allow. Those of us in the arena need to keep reminding the world of this.

I do believe in destiny. I believe Anychild and those of his generation are going to shake this place up and someday make a change. A change so that there will be fewer children on mind altering drugs, less children identified only by the acronym they have been labeled with, more medical insight and support, and more understanding from the world at large. Families will come together to support one another and the dangerous and ignorant Anylookers of this world will be silenced.

Those who are blessed with the white picket fence lives we all want will be forced to peek over that fence and look at the fact that the Anyfamilies of this world are not just collectives of bad children with bad parents, but instead warrior families who have faced unique medical conditions and fought hard for their children's health and well-being.

To the Anyparents who read this book, even though I have likely never met you, we are somehow kindred souls on a shared path. Your pain is my pain, and Anychild's victories, however great or small they end up being, belong to you, too.

On the days when you feel you cannot take one more step forward, be emboldened with the knowing that the path we walk today is paving the way for the Anychildren and Anyparents who will come after us.

Because of what we do today, the Anyfamilies of tomorrow will not have to fight for simple treatments that can change the course of a lifetime.

Sharing Anychild's story is our way of flinging the front door of the PANS world wide open and inviting all of the Anylookers in. That's right, Anylookers. Pull up a chair and take a good long look around. Given one small twist of fate, our house could be your house, too.

Time will show that this house that we live in as an Anyfamily, it is made of brick.

The Anylookers may feel snug in their straw houses for now, but as the biological basis of this illness becomes more and more apparent, the winds of truth are going to huff and they are going to puff and . . .

Well, we all know how that story ends.

EPILOGUE

In 2012, PANS descended into our world and changed everything. Despite this, our story is a happy one. Today, Anychild is indistinguishable from any other child his age. If you were to meet him you would see nothing but a moppy-haired boy who moves through the world way too fast. His bedroom wall is full of trophies, he fights us tooth and nail over homework, and he is a happy, well-adjusted child who is thriving inside and out.

The things that go on behind the scenes to make life 'normal' are invisible to the world. From the outside, you cannot see that our life runs like a machine and that every single day we do what we can to create an immunological fortress around Anychild so that a pathogen does not cross his blood/brain barrier and send us careening into hell. We have prescription bottles of medication lined up in neat rows that are hidden from view, and we have a virtual laundry list of things that we will do at a moment's notice, should a PANS flare show up on the horizon of our world.

Despite the reinforcements that are always in place, life is astonishingly normal. The hard part is knowing that a PANS flare can, at any moment, blow the fuse on our whole system and shut it down. If Anychild gets exposed to strep and it takes hold, his immune system will unwittingly begin to attack his brain. He won't get a fever or a sore throat, or any other outward sign of illness. Anychild will just fall into hell and to the untrained eye, he will look like a bad little boy with equally bad parents. The good part about knowing he has PANS is that we know how to begin climbing out of that hell once the descent starts. The blessing we have that so many other families do not is that we have a PANS-specific medical team to lean toward.

Under the care of the Stanford PANS clinic, Anychild has been able to maintain his strong remission. He has been on daily antibiotics for almost three years and has had no recurrence of strep or any serious PANS flares. He has had mild flares and symptom spikes during several garden-variety illnesses and fevers, but nothing more than a blip on the radar. Compared to the long stretches of hell we experienced at his onset in 2012, intermittently in 2013, and then again in 2015, when he was diagnosed with both strep and Influenza B, these small symptom breakthroughs were easily tolerated.

In early 2016, Anychild complained of a sore throat and spiked a 102-degree fever. His strep screen came back negative, but we could not be certain that it was not strep causing the fever. He quickly began to show the telltale signs of a PANS flare, and acting swiftly, his Stanford care team increased and added to his daily antibiotic dose. Once the fever and signs of infection were gone, they gave Anychild his first 'steroid burst.'

Just like that, within 48 hours, the beasts of anxiety, OCD, sleep disruption, bed wetting, extreme separation anxiety and hyperactivity emerging out of nowhere all lay back down and went to sleep. As his symptoms had begun to ramp up, our team at Stanford wasted no time. Within 24 hours of beginning that steroid burst, Anychild was significantly better. By 48-hours into the burst, he was practically well. He continued to improve over the next five days and his trajectory upward from there has continued.

For over six months after this first steroid burst, he was maintained on a Prednisone dose of 5mg a day. He flourished, perhaps because for the first time in years his brain was finally free of the inflammation that had taken hold. He advanced remarkably in his academic skills during this time and overall became a much happier and healthy child. At the time of this printing we have so far been unsuccessful at being able to taper him off this medication.

No one has to point out to us that it is not ideal for him to be taking daily antibiotics and steroids, but he remains symptom free and he's thriving. When we have attempted to wean him off the steroids, the symptoms of a flare become obvious. As an Anyparent, there is not a day that goes by that I do not worry that we might be making mistakes in our choices for Anychild— but there is no well worn path to follow.

He remains on these daily medications and will until his doctors advise otherwise. We are hopeful that the joyful, happy, healthy boy we have seen these medications uncover will eventually become his set point without the pharmaceutical crutches his wayward immune system so far demands. In the meantime, we work consistently at repairing his gut and detoxing his system from the medications he is on, while we keep our eyes on the horizon of his future.

From the outside, it is easy for people to judge our long term use of antibiotics and steroids and there are more than a few parents and/or doctors who are not shy about sharing their judgment with us. Opinions are free and everyone seems to have one, but for our Anyfamily, who has been sitting in the front row in the world of PANS since 2012, we have learned the hard way that these medications are the lesser of two evils when facing a flare. No one wants their child on long term antibiotics. No parent wants to dole out a steroid to their child daily, but like other PANS families, we go where we must to keep our Anychild well.

Our hope, of course, is to have Anychild off all medications in the future, but at the time of this book's publication (early 2018), under the care of his Stanford medical team, he continues to take daily antibiotics and steroids. He is doing exceedingly well, but healing is a day-by-day journey. The fact that Anychild takes a daily handful of medications *is* worrisome to us, but we are acutely aware of how lucky we have been and how well managed our PANS journey has been compared to what other Anyfamilies have faced. Should Anychild start once again down the pathway of an acute flare, we will do whatever his treatment team advises us to, while remaining mindful of the fact that we are one of the few families—out of hundreds of thousands—who are lucky enough to have a PANS-oriented medical team caring for our child.

I resisted writing this book because I didn't want Anychild to lose his anonymity with the telling of our tale, but the fact that we are fortunate enough to have a bonafide PANS focused medical team is the one thing that has consistently moved me forward toward publication. If we had not been accepted into the Stanford PANS program, I cannot imagine what life might be like today. How other families are surviving without the resources we have been given, I simply cannot fathom.

PANS is estimated to affect one in every 200 children, yet medical resources remain scant. This simply has to change. It is time for the pediatric world of medicine to put the controversy aside and start really listening to Anyfamilies like us. Ours is only one story, but the pain and the struggle that we have faced represents the collective experience of Anyfamilies everywhere.

Our children are burning and the pediatric medical system is looking the other way, refusing to make the paradigm shift that an illness like PANS demands. Accepting that even a small facet of mental illness could be infection or inflammation-based is a concept that truly changes everything, for all of us. A line has been drawn in the sand between physical and mental illness and it appears that the medical community, the pharmaceutical industry, and even society at large have a vested interest in keeping that line clear and tidy. Those of us who live in a world where PANS spews dirt haphazardly on both sides of the line are desperately looking for witnesses, but they continue to be oh, so hard to find.

Asking a complacent medical system to bear witness to a disorder that if seen clearly, could lead to nothing less than a paradigm shift, is a tall order. It will likely remain the work of the Anyfamilies of this world to continue to stand tall and speak our truth.

My hope is that as I end the writing of our story, it will somehow allow me to close the book on what has been a harrowing chapter in our lives. In reality, I am aware that this likely will not be the case, but even if it is, the ways that this illness has changed the fundamental structure of our lives is irreversible.

Yes, PANS has taken from us—it has stolen pieces of our son's childhood that we can never get back—yet it has also given.

What we have gained can best be summed up in that oft-repeated quote whose source I am never quite sure of:

"Be kind, for every man is fighting a battle."

The next time you see a child or a family that does not fit the cookie cutter mold of how things 'should look' in our society, remember this quote, and remember our story. If that out-of-place family looks battle weary and lost, pass this book onto them, or direct them to http://www.shadowsyndromes.com.

As cutting edge pediatric medical research emerges to validate the reality of PANS, let us hope that cures for judgment and ignorance are on the horizon, too.

ANYSTORIES

I delayed the publication of this book because I wanted to share more than just our story. I wanted to show the many faces of PANS.

With Stanford's help, I attempted to consolidate the experiences of other Anyfamilies into this work, but as their stories came in, it quickly became evident that there was no way for me to capture the reality of this illness in short vignettes.

PANS arrives with such varying degrees of severity, and has so many facets to its presentation, that every family's story is a book in itself. *The stories are many and the suffering is vast.*

So, I share here two Anystories, written by Anymoms, in their own words. The first, *On a Wing and a Prayer*, is an Anysaga, a years' long journey deep into the underbelly of PANS. It is told by a true Anymom warrior who has shared her story widely and helped many, including myself, while doing so.

The second, *KB's Timeline*, is simply that, a timeline. It was a real time recording of the first 30 days of an Anychild's descent into hell. I would like to tell you that the descent stopped when the timeline did but it did not. The Anyfamily who shared that timeline resides in a PANS illiterate community and they continually fight for antibiotics for their Anychild. The antibiotics, when they are offered, are given sparingly and begrudgingly.

Two very different Anystories <u>that could be anyone's story.</u>

The world just does not realize this. Yet.

On a Wing and a Prayer

There is a saying that originated out of WWII, "On a wing and a prayer." This sums up our story. A plane came limping back after an attack—this is how I have felt fighting PANS over and over.

The saying is defined to mean, "With only the slightest chance of success," and the key word there is *chance*. When there's little to hold on to, even the slightest bit of hope is what you cling to.

My story actually begins years before my sweet son, who I will call PM, became sick. It begins with my sweet daughter. We had a one-year-old boy so cute, everyone would stop to look at him and say "Aw" as he went by. We also had a five-year-old girl, jaw-dropping in her own right, as well as smart, funny, creative—she loved to make up and sing her own original songs to us, all decked out in whatever fancy (not always matching) clothing she could design.

Life was bliss (well, let's just say it was) until she turned seven and I got the call from my husband. He had taken her to a regular pediatric check-up and the pediatrician had tested her for scoliosis, reporting a positive result. I didn't know what to say. I was shocked . . . we went forward with the xray and specialist visit, to find that she had a near 30 degree curvature in her spine. A curve needing intervention with prosthesis.

I couldn't believe this beautiful girl, an athletic, competitive cheerleader at her tender age, would require a prosthesis. Just the word sent chills down my own spine. And upon arriving at the place that

makes these devices that I know are great for other
people, like ones with no legs, needing a forearm, etc.,
I had no idea she'd be in a prosthetic brace starting
halfway down her buttocks encompassing her entire
trunk up to her armpits for the next three years!!!
This was the worst thing that ever happened to me
(well, and to her). I loved and cherished my children
like nothing I've ever loved before. Just the thought
that she had a deformity almost made me want to
throw up. Well, we'll just do the regular visits and x-
rays and keep on top of the curve. She'll "just" wear
the brace 23 hours per day and we'll see what
happens. Then the worst happened.

At the age of 10 she had her regular xray
checkup. The specialist called while I was in a movie
theatre (a rare outing with two kids!). I vaguely
remember words like "50 degrees, surgery, referral."
I could not hear much else. I immediately called my
husband and sobbed my eyes out in the movie theatre
lobby. People walked by and I just thought, "There
goes another normal person without this horror."
I could barely operate, but my need to get her the
best care possible moved me forward.

I met with world experts. I talked to anyone who
would about the pros/cons of fusion, I blogged like a
maniac, I even watched a spinal fusion surgery
online. In the end, I made the best decision I could
based on what I knew about risk vs. benefit. I could
not allow the potential for her heart and lungs to be
injured. The week before surgery, I saw the hump

that was forming on her right upper back . . . when you love someone, you don't see the blemishes. I almost fainted in the hallway as they wheeled her away. I made the team call me every hour to ensure me they did not impinge on her spinal cord.

When they rolled her out, I hardly knew her face, nor her reconstructed, bedraggled body. There was a rough week in the hospital and a couple at home, but when cheer season came around again in August, a short three months later, she never missed a practice, game or competition. Well, long story short, she turned out to be the poster child of spinal fusion. And, I thought to myself, "Well, nothing worse could possibly happen to us; after all, no family has more than one tragedy." I was wrong.

Little did I know, severe scoliosis, its advocacy, its research, its soul searching, heartwrenching acceptance work I had to do internally, was just preparation for my sweet son, who was now seven-years-old.

We had moved to a small coastal town when PM was one. I decided to return to work after a five year, self employment, stay-at-home mom reprieve. My husband had retired from the Sheriff's department and wanted his turn to be "Mr. Mom" for a while. I obtained a terrific job at a prestigious university in the School of Medicine, where I eventually became an HR Manager and later an operations manager and emergency coordinator for a large science lab, and dad was Dad for a while. Dad decided to return to school a year or two later and he "Dad-ded" and studied for a few years. We were busy but fairly serene when we lost our boy. We were dealing with the aftermath of our sweet daughter's spinal fusion and stress was starting to wind down on the "kid front," until the morning of March 2, 2009, when "aliens" came and took my son's brain.

PM became quite ill very suddenly at the age of seven. He showed sudden symptoms which appeared overnight, including: violence, rage, aggression, drooling, speech impediments, age regression, hallucinations, a strange grin on his face, and we found him pulling up flooring and stabbing our office door with a knife in the middle of the night. Had the stress of his sister's issues gotten to him and turned him into a demonic serial killer?

We went to the ER where he then calmed. They proceeded to tell us he was probably just having a temper tantrum. I tried to explain: They would not listen. We went home and he began to tear his room apart wildly, flailing, barking like a dog on all fours. I knew we had to go back to ER but I waited. I got my camera.

He was hospitalized 50 times and was forcibly removed by Sheriffs on a "5150" 72-hour hold (for his safety and the safety of others) a total of 26 times, both from my home and even twice from a level fourteen residential facility which was equipped for restraint and treatment—that's how severe he was.

The illness hit so sudden and was so extreme, we and the doctors didn't know what to do. Facility after facility would say things like we must be parenting him wrong, try this or try that: he's schizophrenic, bipolar, ODD, ADD, OCD, autistic, etc. They would even accuse us of child abuse, as his behaviors were those of an abused child and he was covered in bruises due to his critically low platelets.

There is no quick way to describe what our family went through. However, some illustrations may be useful:

- My ten-year-old daughter would have to call 911 while I restrained him.
- My ex-Sheriff husband would have trouble keeping him from hurting himself.
- We were hyper-vigilant and scared that at any time he could have an episode and cause physical and property destruction.
- He would jump from moving cars.
- He would bark like a dog and flop around on his knees.
- He experienced audio and visual hallucinations.
- He tried pulling his teeth out.
- He stabbed the kitchen door with a knife in the middle of the night over and over.
- He injured an EMT, requiring stitches.

- He ransacked a couple homes near EMQ in Los Gatos. It was very scary.

We experienced a nonstop flood of psychiatrists, medical doctors, nurses, interns, school officials, county mental health professionals, police, sheriffs, EMTs, paramedics, and fireman that found it hard to believe a child so small and so young could be this difficult to control and so completely out of his mind.

Over a period of about a year and a half he was placed in the San Mateo, San Francisco, and Santa Clara County Psych units, St. Helena in Vallejo, EMQ in Los Gatos, Rebekah's in Gilroy, and many hospital emergency rooms and pediatric units throughout the Bay Area, even one as far as Sacramento due to the shortage of adolescent facilities.

Eventually, it was necessary for him to live in a residential facility as his behaviors could no longer be controlled safely from the home. These hospitalizations were a hardship on the family, but they were also a hardship on PM since the psychiatrists weren't familiar with the medical aspects of his disorder, and couldn't treat that piece of the puzzle. I had to shuttle information constantly between hospital staff, psychiatrists, psychologists, and the medical doctors and specialists.

In these units, my son who had never been exposed to neglect, abuse or violence, was around disturbing behaviors and stories which added to his personal stress. It was also quite difficult to provide appropriate family support for this little seven-year-old when the facilities were often far away. For example, St. Helena in Vallejo was closed to visitors at 7:30 pm; if I left work at 5:00 pm in traffic from Palo Alto, I would have about a half hour to see him and sometimes I wouldn't get to see him at all if there was a violent child and the unit was on lockdown.

Fortunately, I was working around some great minds at Stanford in Pediatrics and my Division Chief felt these were symptoms of inflammation or vasculitis in his brain. I was referred to Lucile Packard's Children's Rheumatology Department where dozens of tests were sent to labs all over the country looking for answers.

He had weekly blood draws, sometimes daily when his platelets were critically low. He had MRIs, lumbar punctures, EEG, seizure and sleep studies, etc. You never want an abnormal test result for your child until you are endlessly searching without answers and feel so helpless. Eventually, a test came back positive and my son's particular "brand" of PANS is called "antiphospholipid syndrome."

PANS or Pediatric Acute Neuro-psychiatric Syndrome is an umbrella that includes a number of illnesses and/or infectious agents that cause this disease pattern. It is believed that this, along with a genetic predisposition, may be the culprits. Having a diagnosis allowed us to aggressively treat PM with chemotherapy, in order to shut down his immune system and interrupt the disease process causing the brain inflammation and the frightening behaviors.

He continues chemotherapy today along with a cocktail of psychiatric medications. His illness is considered to be in a period of acquiescence while on medication. We hope to try taking him off the potentially harmful chemo in the near future; however, we believe PANS is similar to other autoimmune disorders like Lupus, and will be relapsing/remitting throughout his lifetime.

In closing, I run a parent support group for PANS parents at Stanford and I talk with many other PANS parents and patients via social media. There are so many cases out there—even more as awareness increases with diagnosis and treatment protocols being developed.

KB's 30-Day Timeline

By history KB was a developmentally normal healthy five-year-old girl. No history of anything even remotely suggestive of the symptom set that arrived on November 30th.

- **Nov 30th** Totally different kid. Came home from school saying I think I behaved, but I don't know if I did or not. Confessions about things that had happened over the last couple of months at school that were super insignificant. Didn't realize what was going on, so had her write a letter to her teacher apologizing for her behavior. Horrible time concentrating to do homework that is normally very easy for her.

• **Thursday Dec 3rd** Called pediatrician to seek advice. She suspected trauma and asked us to look into it.

• **Saturday Dec 5th** Called pediatrician at Pediatric Urgent care after hearing KB say that her brain was telling her that she hates her mom. Pediatrician said there wasn't anything she could do for us with the exception of examining her physically and doing a strep test to check for strep/PANDAS. Said she didn't think it was PANDAS due to it being very rare. Asked if she could've gotten into anyone's meds. Said to call Monday morning and schedule an appt if not better by then.

• **Throughout weekend** KB would come to me crying saying, "My brain keeps telling me bad things and keeps telling me to misbehave and I don't know what to do. My brain keeps telling me that I hate my mom." Asked if she hated her mom or loved her mom and she said she didn't know. Told her to try to tell her brain that she loves her mom when it tries to tell her that she hates her and she said she did, but that it didn't work. Said her brain told her, "To kill her Dad."

• **Monday Dec 7th** Brought KB into pediatrician's office. Pediatrician tried to offer advice with some of her behaviors. Quick strep test negative, but question if it was a good swab as KB did not come close to gagging. MD said she wanted to run labs to check thyroid. I asked if we could check anti-strep titer while we were doing blood work. She said "Yes, might as well since we're already getting all he-be-gee-bee." I also asked for antibiotics as risk is low to see if improvement in symptoms. She agreed.

• **Tuesday Dec 8th** had blood work done. Started antibiotics (amoxicillin 250mg, 3x/day) that evening. Wednesday Dec 9th got blood work back with positive anti-strep titer (413 with norm range 0-200).

• **After about three days** on ABX, started returning back to her normal self with almost complete resolution of symptoms by end of 10-day course.

• **After three days without ABX**, symptoms started to return. Tried to call pediatricians office to resume ABX but it was the Wednesday before Christmas and the doctor was not in the office. All other providers in the practice refused to help us. Struggled through the week/weekend. Lots of aggression toward her brother that was beyond what is normal for her, crazy amounts of activity (hyperactivity probably the best way to describe it. It wasn't just a lot of activity, it was crazy activity). Continued with intrusive thoughts, confessions, self doubt. Started pulling out her hair, cutting her nails and skin around her nails really short to the point that she would bleed. Had to hide the nail clippers. Also started with cleanliness issues. Asked us to wipe her when she was previously wiping herself. Would say things like, "I washed my hands 3x at grandma and grandpa's but they still didn't feel clean," or "I got out of the shower but had to get back in because I didn't feel like I was clean enough."

• **Called Pediatrician first thing Monday** morning following the Christmas holiday weekend. She said there wasn't anymore she could do for us. Suggested psychiatrist referral for SSRI prescription. Also said she would refer us to Stanford PANDAS clinic. Told her I didn't think we could get in.

• **Pediatrician called back shortly after** and said that she wouldn't be able to get us into Stanford PANDAS clinic, but Stanford doc said we never should've stopped antibiotics and that when kiddos do that, it becomes hard to recapture them. The doctor apologized and said she didn't know any differently. Said that we would treat aggressively going forward. Started on two ABX (Zithromax and amoxicillin) as well as five day burst of steroids. Also wanted to order brain MRI.

- **Started new meds on 12/28.**
- **Had brain MRI on 12/30.**

-End of the first thirty days of PANS.

OUR STORY, YOUR STORY, ANY STORY

These two Anystories are just infinitesimal glimpses of the PANS stories that the Anyfamilies of this world all tell.

Every week on the private PANS Facebook page I still peruse daily, there will be a new mother introducing herself hesitantly with some variation of the statement: "I am new to this group . . . " and what follows will be a harrowing account of a classic PANS onset that will rock every seasoned Anyparent who reads it. It brings it all back when we witness another Anyparent going down the rabbit hole, a parent who does not yet know that her life has taken an off ramp to hell, and that this is not just a passing phase, and that there are no quick, easy answers.

Worst of all, they do not yet know that there are no doctors to care for their children. When you begin this journey, it is inconceivable to think that you will not be able to find medical care: not at onset, not six months in, sometimes not ever. And these newly baptized parents do not yet realize that the more pronounced their child's illness becomes and the more desperately they seek help, the more they will be shunned and questioned, and the more isolating and futile the fight will become.

These neophyte parents have not yet learned that in order to fight PANS you have to get quiet. They do not yet see that PANS is a battle that must be fought underground. They do not yet know that the Facebook group they have just reached out to will likely become their lifeline, or that the Anyparents they will meet there will become some of their closest confidantes.

Eventually, as the newness wears off and they buckle their seatbelts for the long haul, they too will become well seasoned PANS parents. Someday in the future they will find themselves rocked when they read a Facebook post that a desperate parent is making at their child's onset. They will feel all of the things that I have just described, and they will likely reach out to that parent and extend some bit of hard earned wisdom they have gained on the journey.

PANS is like a horrible circle dance, one that no one ever wants to enter into. But I have learned that if we are called to the dance, the one grace that we are given is that Anyparents take care of one another. For now, finding and connecting with other

Anyparents is a primary way many of us make our way through.

I can tell you as an Anymom who is years into this journey, the predictability of it all is sickening, but that predictability has created a sense of community among Anyparents that is truly changing lives and making a difference. It will, of course, be up to science and research to answer the big questions about PANS, but in the meantime, the grassroots wisdom that is forming among Anyparents is proving to be big medicine.

May this book and our story add to this wealth of grassroots wisdom and help bring the reality of PANS out of the shadows and into the light of day.

GIVING BACK

If you are an Anyfamily and have purchased a print copy of this book, know that 20% of the net proceeds of every book purchased will go to a PANS research/ treatment program. Though the number of noteworthy PANS-affiliated research and treatment programs continues to grow, our donations will go to: **The Stanford PANS Clinic and Research Fund.** As a family we also donate to **The PANDAS/PANS Institute.** These programs represent different sides of the same coin: Stanford provides patient care, and conducts state of the art academic and clinical research that is published in peer reviewed journals, while the PANDAS/PANS Institute provides direct patient care, and conducts clinical research that is not constrained by an academic affiliation.

These programs and their leaders (**Dr. Jennifer Frankovich** with **Stanford** and **Dr. Rosario Trifiletti** with the **PANDAS/PANS Institute**) are dear to our hearts. When we came to them as medical refugees, they stepped up to offer us a homeland.

The care and validation they have provided has been instrumental in healing more than just Anychild's immune system.

RESOURCES

Please note this is only a partial listing of resources available and any web addresses and blog addresses offered are subject to change.

WEBSITES AND ORGANIZATIONS

http://www.shadowsyndromes.com
http://www.stanfordchildrens.org/en/service/pans-pandas
http://www.pandasinstitute.org
http://www.pandasnetwork.org
http://www.pandasppn.org
http://www.latitudes.org
http://www.nepans.org
http://www.NIMH.nih.gov
http://www.pas.care
http://www.Midwestpandas.com
http://www.kids.iocdf.org
http://www.aealliance.org
http://www.moleculeralabs.com

INTERNATIONAL WEBSITES AND ORGANIZATIONS

CANADA
www.pandascanada.wix.com/pandascanada

ITALY

www.pandasitalia.it

SWEDEN
www.panspandas.se

BLOGS

NEPANS Blog
http://www.nepans.org/nepansblog

PANS Life
http://www.panslife.com

PANDAS Sucks
https://www.pandassucks.com

The PANDAS Puzzle
http://www.thepandaspuzzle.com

The Dreaming PANDA
http://www.thedreamingpanda.wordpress.com

Life with PANDAS
http://www.lifewithpandas.wordress.org

Three with ADHD
http://www.3withadhd.com

Biomed Heals
http://www.biomedheals.com

BOOKS

Saving Sammy: A Mother's Fight to Cure Her Son's OCD
By Beth Alison Maloney

Childhood Interrupted: The Complete Guide to PANDAS and PANS
By Beth Alison Maloney

Brain on Fire: My Month of Madness
By Susannah Cahalan

In A Pickle Over PANDAS
By Melanie S. Weiss

PANS, CANS, and Automobiles: A Comprehensive Reference Guide for Helping Students with PANDAS and PANS
By Jamie Candelaria Greene

Pandas and Pans in School Settings
By Patricia Rice Doran and Diana Pohlman

FACEBOOK

There are many regional, national, and international groups out there. Search for what you need. Some are Closed/Private Parents groups, some are Causes and Advocacy.

PANDAS Resource Network
P.A.N.D.A.S. Network
PANDAS Physicians Network
"Parents" of kids with PANDAS/PITANDS/PANS
Homeopathy for Autism, PANDAS/PANS
Oils for PANDAS
PANDAS A Real Life Case of Jekyll and Hyde
Stanford Area PANS Parents Support Group

AUDIO-VISUAL & EDUCATIONAL RESOURCES FOR PARENTS, CAREGIVERS & PROVIDERS
www.Mykidisnotcrazy.com
This is a documentary about PANS/PANDAS featuring some of today's top physicians and researchers. It will be available on DVD in 2017.

Moleculara LABS and Cunningham Panel video

There are videos on YouTube created by both parents and providers. There are individual stories, physicians citing research, and recordings of provider presentations from regional, national, and international conferences. Search for them.

Index

A

Abrupt, 15, 75
Abuse, 92,
    113–119, 131,
    161, 179
ABX, 204, 206
Accusations,
    114, 118, 131,
    178
ache, 48, 84
Acronym, 31,
    44, 91, 133,
    138, 141–142,
    182, 184
Acute, 6, 12, 21,
    40, 56, 66,
    82–83, 101,
    107, 117, 127,
    132, 142, 144,
    155, 159, 164,
    166, 177, 191

ADHD, 48, 106,
    135, 141, 182,
    210
admission, 74,
    81, 87, 95,
    101, 182
adrenal, 61–62
Advil, 64, 69–70,
    172
Advocacy, 116,
    121, 128, 181,
    197, 212
AE, 133, 144
Afflict, 7, 49, 60,
    142, 164–165
Aggression, 54,
    198, 204, 206
Allegations, 116,
    179
Allele, 23,
    154–156
allergic, 120,

Index

Index

Index

Index

Index

Index

Index

E

Index

Index

Index

147–156, 158,
173–174

glutened, 151

H

handwriting, 135
Harvard, 49
headache, 70
heal, 6, 17, 23,
    87, 100–102,
    120, 128, 131,
    141, 145–149,
    156, 161, 169,
    191, 211
heart, 46, 77,
    115, 197
hemolytic, 134
Herpes, 133, 159
heterodimer, 154
HHV, 39, 133,
    159–160
HLA, 23, 154
homeopath,
    157, 212
Hospital, 11,

107, 111,
113–114, 121,
129, 183, 198
hydrated, 69,
    176
hygienist, 59, 65
hyperactive, 33,
    36, 42, 54, 82,
    93, 122,
    134–135, 141,
    166, 176–177,
    182, 189, 205
hypervigilant,
    176
hypothesis, 27,
    31, 138

I

ibuprofen,
    172–173
IED, 141, 182
IgA, 21, 156, 158
IgE, 158
Igenex, 158
IgG, 21, 156,

Index

Index

156

intravenous, 44,
138–139

intrusive, 13,
162, 205

involuntary, 42,
48

irritability, 126,
135, 167

irritating, 178

IV, 73, 75–76,
80, 97–98, 100

IVIG, 44,
137–139

J

joint, 66, 122,
127, 135–136

judged, 128, 131

judgment, 4,
113, 117, 190,
193

K

Kinase, 161

kindergarten, 5,
7, 170

L

lab, 39, 61, 78,
99, 119, 197

Laboratories, 23

laboratory, 153,
155, 158

labs, 62, 73–74,
76, 81–82, 85,
106, 158, 160,
204, 212

lactic, 148

laundry, 103,
106, 187

LDN, 63

leukocyte, 154

limbs, 82

Limp, 122, 195

Index

Index

Nucleus, 52
Nutrition, 44,
    120, 150, 158,
    168

O

Obligate, 53
obsessed, 33
obsessions, 65,
    161–162
obsessive, 36,
    42, 51, 55,
    132, 134, 141,
    161, 178, 182
OCD, 33, 42,
    55–56, 106,
    132, 135, 141,
    161–162, 164,
    182, 189, 211
onset, 14–16,
    18, 20, 22, 33,
    40–41, 43–44,
    56, 88, 120,
    132, 134–135,
    139–141,

143–144, 147,
149, 156, 160,
162–166, 171,
177, 188,
206–207
openly, 116, 119
Oppositional,
    14, 141, 182
organism, 136
overprotective,
    54, 178

P

pain, 4, 7, 27,
    66, 71, 81, 88,
    102, 127, 135,
    181, 185, 191
paranoia, 110
paranoid, 105,
    109
Parvovirus, 159
pathogen, 187
pathways, 18,
    136, 145, 168,
    171, 191

Index

Index

120, 141,
165–166, 182
prophylactic, 64
Protective, 48,
55, 91–92
provider, 43–44,
69, 113–114,
204, 212
Psychiatirc, 33
psychiatric,
10–11, 16, 20,
31, 33, 40,
43–44, 48–49,
130, 132,
140–145, 147,
149, 182–183
psychiatrist, 20,
205
psychiatry, 33,
48
psychology, 14
psychosis, 22,
147
psychotropic,
50, 144, 146
PTSD, 174, 177
pupils, 32–33

R

rage, 8, 10,
12–13, 19,
23–24, 26–30,
32–33, 36–37,
52, 59, 78, 83,
99, 103, 136,
146, 162,
164–165, 198
ranting, 30
Rapp, 157
reactive, 51, 90,
136, 150, 153,
155
reference, 3, 211
referral, 3, 10,
16, 38, 57, 62,
88, 92, 101,
123, 196, 205
refusal, 4, 89,
109–110, 163,
192, 204
regression, 42,
143–144, 198
relationship, 25,
121
relationships,

Index

Index

Index

Index

Index

Index

Index

walker,
100–102, 112
walking, 4, 32,
163, 179
watching, 12,
36, 46, 51, 71,
86, 103, 121,
125, 176
wheat, 21–22,
155, 163

Zithromax, 206

xray, 195–196

Y

Yale, 34, 49
Yasko, 169
yeast, 45

Made in the USA
San Bernardino, CA
05 February 2019